GOD HAD OTHER PLANS

HEATHER D. NELSON

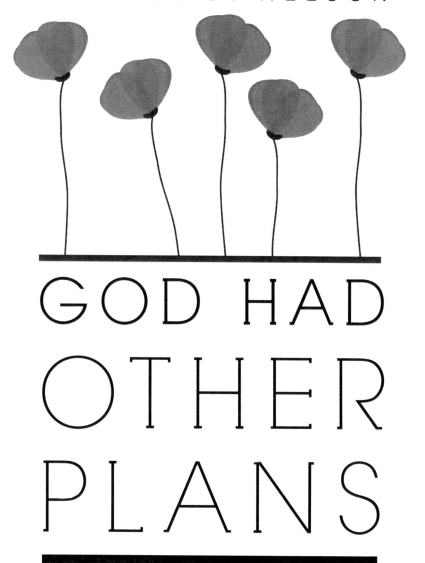

GOD HAD OTHER PLANS

**KEEPING FAITH THROUGH
PREGNANCY LOSS AND INFERTILITY**

Tate Publishing & Enterprises

Published by Tate Publishing & Enterprises, LLC
127 E. Trade Center Terrace | Mustang, Oklahoma 73064 USA
1.888.361.9473 | www.tatepublishing.com

Tate Publishing is committed to excellence in the publishing industry. The company reflects the philosophy established by the founders, based on Psalm 68:11,
"The Lord gave the word and great was the company of those who published it."

Book design copyright © 2010 by Tate Publishing, LLC. All rights reserved.
Cover design by Lauran Levy
Interior design by Joel Uber

Published in the United States of America

ISBN: 978-1-61739-241-2
1. Biography & Autobiography, Personal Memoirs
2. Biography & Autobiography, Women
10.10.20

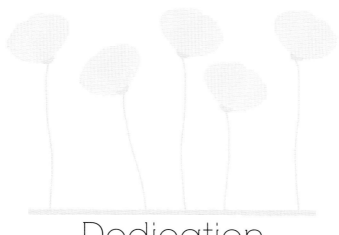

Dedication

To my husband Kevin.

You are absolutely, without fail, my rock in this life. Your unwavering faith and constancy have always been a corner stone for me. My world is infinitely better because you are in it. Olive juice more today and every day… forever.

And now it's in print… beat that!

And to my precious angel-baby, Peanut.

Your life was short-lived but powerful. May the love in our hearts for you forever bring about love and understanding in others.

Mommy and Daddy love you forever.

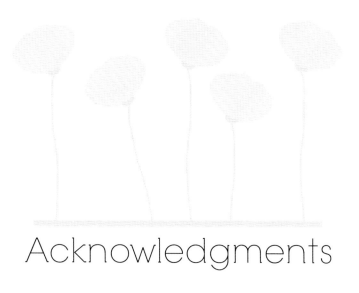

Acknowledgments

It goes without saying that this book would not exist if not for the will of God and the love and support of my husband so top billing on my list of people to thank goes to them. God inspired me to use our struggles as a tool *to hopefully help* others. Blessing me as only He can, God gave me the ultimate in support in my husband, Kevin, who has put me back together more times than I care to admit.

And of course, what would this book be without the constant care and guidance of my incredible team of doctors who cared for me and my little family over a period of nearly three years. A special thank you goes out to Dr. Hayes, Dr. Greer, and Dr. Slater. Oh yeah, and thanks Dr. Agrussa too for putting me on bed rest and making me finish this book! Through our entire infertility journey, the support we received from our church family was constant. The prayer was sustaining and certainly the occasional cards of concern were well-timed and well-received. An extra note of gratitude should be given to The Mogfords, The Davis,' The Benzyls, The McMillans, The Barnes, and The Jenkins. Be it a refuge to hide out for a time or a shoulder to cry on, they offered them equally and with full hearts. We are forever grateful.

Last, but never least, to my wonderful mother-in-law. Despite my constant protestations, I did finally take your advice and start writing, first to Peanut, then in journals and online support forums. Your suggestions helped spark this urge in me to grow past myself and it has, hopefully, led to me helping others.

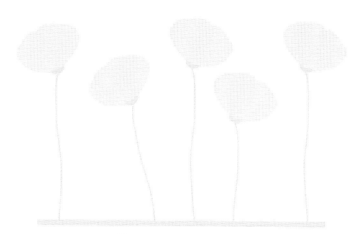

Contents

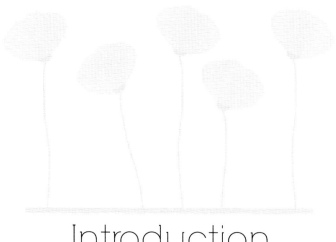

Introduction

This is an excerpt from my first journal entry ever:

March 20, 2008

Here I sit. Having had the worst year of my life in 2007. I now stare down the barrel of 2008 with a very bleak outlook and no hope that the light at the end of the tunnel is not just bringin' an oncoming freight train of pain.

My faith is shaken; I'm totally pessimistic and feel utterly defeated. My family cannot relate, nor can our friends, and I feel like I have no one to talk to. Sadly, people who think they are well-meaning are actually really hurtful in the things they say. Granted if they knew more, they'd make different choices, but I simply do not feel safe enough to put myself out there anymore and explain anything, or even ask for what I need. This is personal and hard, the people in my life can be judgmental. Why do people assume I should be "okay" about the miscarriage? Why do people make remarks like, "You're so pessimistic" when I express concern for our future attempts at a family? I want to scream at them, "Well duh, I've been trying to have a baby for over a year and have been told I've got a snowball's chance in hell at it, and the one pregnancy I did get netted me a dead baby and a horrid D & C procedure—I'm entitled to a little pessimism!"

But I will not, I never do. I know in my heart they mean well and I am just in a bad place emotionally, I will do what I always do. I retreat and hide and I do not talk to them about it. I have some people in my life who are very supportive, but even they cannot totally relate, and I often feel like some of them feel encouraged to "counsel" me for their own feel-good gain. How's that for a horrible outlook on life? Am I awful or what?

I love my husband unendingly. He's amazingly supportive through all this and has never complained about my ups and downs, but I cannot lean on him 100 percent of the time or he'll get burned out too. I need someone—anyone—who's been there to just give me some freakin' hope that I'll survive all this and end up with what I want so very badly.

To be fair, this book is more a published cathartic rant on my struggles of infertility, as well as a personal tracking of the ups and downs that infertility and pregnancy loss put me through. Granted, as I sit here and write this book, I can fully and successfully say I have *been there* and *done that* and been out the other side of it all, relatively unscathed. But truth be told, survival changes nothing on the scars that infertility leaves behind on your heart. Infertility is a deeply personal and potentially life-sucking struggle that alters your perception of everything in an instant. Within a short six-month period, I went from goal focused and ignorantly blissful to depressed and dumbstruck and lost. And in the middle of all this, where was God?

For over a year before writing this book, I felt compelled to start journaling my experience and trying to learn and cope with my ordeal. But soon thereafter, I started feeling the call to write a sort of "self-help" book to help other couples deal with infertility. About two months into that I realized: who the heck am I to *self-help* anyone? I'm a mess and have no business guiding others! Yet still, I felt like a book was in order, but what kind of book became the question. Slowly over time (two-plus years to be exact) I shaped the idea that what would have *most* helped me during my struggle was just knowing other couples who had walked where we were walking, or rather, other couples who had survived the waters that we were then drowning in. Simply knowing I was not alone, crazy, and thoroughly abandoned in society would have been the biggest blessing I could have asked for. And so this book was born. To share all our ups and downs, and with them all how we kept our marriage intact along with our faith and came out stronger on the other side in both!

It is the story of one insignificant Christian couple's road to family life with incredible obstacles, insane humor, and all the tears, bliss, peace, pain, and joy that came along with it.

To be sure, my life has grown and changed through and beyond infertility and pregnancy loss to other beautiful and wondrous things. However, to date, nothing has shaped me more as a woman. Do I believe God personally chose to sit up on His cloud and smite my efforts to be a mother as to somehow shape me? Absolutely not, at least not now. But I do believe, *strongly*, that God used this time in such a way to reach me that I might never have been reached otherwise. As Beth Moore quoted one time, "Perhaps [I] am not picked on…but rather [I] have been picked out," and here is the real kicker—*I'm grateful.* I am thankful for what God has taught me and grateful for the way this journey has tempered my heart, strengthened my marriage, and stretched me to be more than I was before. My only aspiration now is that I can continue to use this precious gift God has given me as a tool to hopefully help some other couple out there who is sitting in their home, crying, and asking God, "Why?"

Hopefully this book will be an opportunity for some other couple to finally find that balance in both understanding their current baby-making struggles, and resolving that their faith and marriage can and should be unshakable throughout it. At the very least, maybe this will offer a brief glance for any friends and family members of someone struggling. A window—if you will—into the infertility and pregnancy loss world.

From Woo-Hoo to Whoa

My memory of that first day of our long journey to a family is pristine in my mind—that wonderful, glorious day. The day when my husband, Kevin, and I finally agreed it was time to start a family. Or, as I like to joke in my more crude moments, to take the goalie out of the net and shoot to score. We had been married for a year and a half (as was the previously agreed on time to wait) but more than that, we both deemed it was the *right* time. It was a weird but wonderful moment as we sat in our living room together talking, and both of us simultaneously felt that *this* was the right time. I felt that our concurrent good feelings were a sign from God that we were on the right track. And if God agreed, then, *for sure*, this would be a quick process. We talked about adoption, which I always loved the idea of, but in the end both of us agreed we wanted a biological child of our very own. We ceremoniously tossed my birth control pills in the trash and proceeded to celebrate our decision with some serious sheet frolicking. As I rested my head on the pillow that night, and nearly every night thereafter, I prayed to God. I thanked God for such a loving, wonderful husband and I asked him to bless us with *our* baby and fashion for us, at last, a family.

As a newlywed who felt our honeymoon was bliss, I was not prepared for the rush that came over my husband and I. As I would learn, there is no greater aphrodisiac than a committed, loving couple deciding to *try* for a baby. I was suddenly a ravenous woman and my man was *all too glad* to oblige me, regardless of the time of day or night or frequency, etc. We were no longer being together for recreational value. Now we were *making a baby*, and that higher calling reached me in ways I could not have fathomed. For a good two months, life was grand. Bliss even! I charted and tracked and calculated and timed and organized it all into a handy notebook that I carried around with me. I even plotted ways to pounce on my husband when the time was right, and he enjoyed the perceived spontaneity of it all. I was *planning* our family right down to calculating hopeful due dates each month and dreaming of what each new day would bring. Each week I would envision what our new due date would be, and how that time of the year would make for a good birthday for our child. Then, of course, I would sit around and daydream about what our baby would look like. It would be a boy first, I had decided, then maybe later a girl. The boy would have his daddy's eyes and broad shoulders and quiet strength. Our daughter would have my dark hair and artistic side. They would both be utter geniuses of course, and we would be the picture of perfection as our family grew through the years. *Sigh.* My plans were perfect. Then, things changed.

Enter Dr. Hayes

I had seen my primary care doctor before we began trying to conceive, and I mentioned what our plans were. He said that he and his wife had needed a little help having a baby, and suggested that I proactively track my cycles using my basal body temperature (BBT) each month. Looking back I can see that God placed the right person in my life at *just* the right time. This little passing advice saved me hoards of time. Within two months of tracking I realized my cycles were a little wonky and by the third month, I was pretty sure I was not even ovulating on a normal schedule. This was slightly disappointing to me, but not entirely unexpected given my health history. I dutifully informed my OB-GYN, Dr. Hayes, and she looked over all my charts and promptly announced that

I had indeed rejoined the ranks of the Polycystic Ovarian Syndromer's out there. In fact, I was anovulatory which is a fancy word for someone who does not ovulate in a regular manner or who has a jacked up luteal phase. I was not surprised by this but it was still a bit of a bummer. I thought that my big efforts to lose weight and be healthier prior to this time would have slapped my PCOS into a remission of sorts, and I was discouraged to find out that it never goes away, *ever*. We had only been trying since November 2006 and as of February 2007; we were already in Dr. Hayes' office discussing options. She suggested we try Metformin, at 1500mg per day, to get my body more healthy. She said it would help my insulin resistance, be better for my heart, and put me in a healthier place all around. As a side effect it *could* help with my ovulation as well, so we might as well do this step first and see if it helps to kick start things more naturally. She went on to say that, *if* nothing improved by April we'd move on to more assistance as needed, including Clomid to force ovulation.

I was less than thrilled with *her* plan. I had charts; I had *plans* of my own! I had tracked, organized, and even documented all my ovulatory information into handy Microsoft Excel charts and graphs. I had even prayed fervently and received what I felt was sure confirmation from God that I was on the right path. Surely she could *see* how serious I was about having a baby *right now*. Who cares about my personal health, I wanted a baby, thank you very much! Moreover, if we did not hurry, my original plan for a winter baby would be whisked away and I would have to plan for another due date. Did Dr. Hayes not see how much her, "wait and see" approach was cramping my style?!?

My dutiful husband, who was there at this fateful appointment, and heard the alarming heart attack statistics that accompany PCOS, wholeheartedly agreed with the doctor that my personal health and safety came first, and the baby-making could stand to wait a few more months. That traitor.

Fine, I thought. *I am outnumbered, I guess I will take the Metformin, continue tracking and charting and planning and see what happens while being the dutiful patient. It is only another three months and we have some traveling to do for my dear cousin's wedding after all. Fine... no big deal... whatever.* The good attitude was practically pouring out of me at this point.

As a good wife and patient, I did everything within my power to make Metformin the winning punch we needed. I continued to pray nightly for God to give us *our* baby. I took my pills each day as prescribed, dealt with any minor, if not gross, side effects that Metformin caused, and only noticed a *slight* drop in my "sheet music" enthusiasm with my husband. As the time passed between February and April, I noticed a few good things about the medication, mainly a reduction in other PCOS related symptoms I had been otherwise ignoring. However, as April came around I still had only ovulated once in a three-month period. I felt somewhat vindicated when I next saw Dr. Hayes and defiantly said, "See, not all's well in fertile-ville, so *gimme the good drugs.*" I was practically sticking my tongue out and stomping my foot like a willful child. Dr. Hayes and my husband agreed that it was time for more aggressive measures and I was given the instructions and prescription I needed to officially re-begin our baby-making efforts with the help of both Metformin and Clomid. As I left that fateful visit with Dr. Hayes, I could almost hear the angelic hallelujah chorus.

I laugh now thinking of how I viewed Clomid as "more aggressive measures." *Man alive,* was I clueless about how advanced medical science has come in this area!

Dr. Hayes said that Clomid is a very inexpensive drug option that often works well in conjunction with Metformin, and is a great place to start for women who are anovulatory and who have PCOS struggles. I was to take that for five days, then test for ovulation using these handy kits you buy at the drugstore. How easy was that? Then, when the little pee stick lights up that I'm ovulating, Kevin and I "do the deed." Not only could I stop tracking my stupid BBT (which was utter torture by then), but I could just pee on a stick to be 100 percent sure of ovulation; this should be a slam dunk now. Baby Town, here I come! In my mind, I was already recalculating proposed due dates and planning out our lives with what I was sure was our future child, and *all* of this while still sitting on the exam table in Dr. Hayes' office. It's *amazing* how quickly my mind can work when I am truly passionate for something. However, Dr.

Hayes interrupted my daydream by interjecting a little precaution. She told me that *just* to make sure they do not put me through any unnecessary medication, we should do a quick semen analysis on my husband. It was supposed to be simply a matter of standard practice and precaution. It was said to be quick, painless, cheap, and would rule out any problems with him so we could barrel forward 100 percent confident in our direction. As long as it did not interfere with my plans I was on board. It was cheap and painless which put Kevin on board too. At that final agreement, we made the necessary appointments and prepared to meet the Urologist, Dr. Greer.

Enter Dr. Greer

Dr. Greer was nice enough as far as doctors go. He was timely in his appointments, explanatory in what he was going to do, and even addressed any questions my husband and I had. He explained what they would be looking for and what all tests they would run, etc. As a side note to wives out there, I found this process utterly hysterical. I mean seriously, I hop into stirrups at *least* once a year, if not more, and try to find a happy place while some doctor that I am *paying* proceeds to invade my nether regions in ways that seriously violate all the "stranger danger" rules I was given growing up. When the urologist proposed that my husband needed a quick "physical exam" to ensure all his parts were where they needed to be, Kevin's face turned red up to his ears and it was all I could do to maintain my calm and leave the room without bursting into maniacal laughter. And again, when that exam was over and the young female receptionist at Dr. Greer's office sent us home with a paper bag and plastic cup (with instructions), my husband turned beet-red with embarrassment and the giggles bubbled up and leaked out a little. I was still planning and plotting our future baby's due date 100 percent sure that we would be pregnant in no time flat. I felt confident that all of this was a waste of our time, but it sure was nice of Dr. Hayes to be cautious and thorough. Each night, I would lay my head on my pillow and thank God for a loving husband and ask Him to bless us with *our* baby.

When the date came for us to send the "man sample" to Dr. Greer, I tried to sound dignified and respectful as I gently and softly asked my loving husband if he needed any help in accomplishing his task. He gave me a *firm* NO and then went upstairs, alone, and took care of his husbandly duties as prescribed by Dr. Greer's instruction sheet. I remained downstairs with the paper bag in hand, paperwork all filled out, so we could rush the collection to Dr. Greer in time for the analysis to be completed. And by rush I mean speed slightly over the posted limits and pray for good traffic and no construction zones. As it turns out…man samples are very time sensitive and if you arrive too late all your work goes, quite literally, down the drain! Lord knows my husband had made it clear that he did *not* want to endure this embarrassment *in* the actual office, so we needed to seriously hustle. Once our delivery was made, Dr. Greer told us we would get the results from Dr. Hayes. We waited and I prayed for a quick turnaround in results and, of course, for God to bless us with *our* baby. In the meantime, my cycle was coming around and I filled my prescription for Clomid thus preparing myself for the baby-making festivities to come. I envisioned how beautiful our little baby boy would look and even started to envision myself in fall fashion maternity clothes. Then, the truly unexpected happened.

It was a Friday afternoon and I was getting ready to be picked up by some friends to go on a weekend ladies retreat with our church. We were going to a cute little town about two hours up in the mountains from us. I was never a "sing-a-long-hug-a-tree-to-bond-retreat" type of person, but was begged and bribed into going and was actually beginning to look forward to the getaway. Besides, according to my charts, I was to begin the first round of Clomid upon my return and we could try for a baby shortly after that. That made this retreat my final hurrah before I became a mother… yippee. What was not to love about a ladies retreat?

Around 1:00 p.m., my phone rang and it was Dr. Hayes. Let me emphasize that it was not Dr. Hayes' nurse or one of Dr. Hayes' office staff… but actually Dr. Hayes. I should have known right then that something was up but I was oblivious, as usual. I expected her to tell me all was fine and we could begin the Clomid and "baby-dancing" as soon as I returned from my retreat. But alas, she was not calling to be so kind. She told me very calmly that there was a problem with the semen analysis. Granted, she told me in very professional and technical terms, but basically, my brain went a little foggy so the details were a bit lost on me. As I understood things, my husband had some motility issues and some morphology issues and some viscosity issues to round it all out. Or, in more crude but understandable terms, his boys were lazy, half of them were misshapen, and that made the good ones rather stuck and ineffective. I asked her what that meant and she said, "You should not start the Clomid this next cycle. This is a bigger problem that we need to deal with before moving forward. You need to go see Dr. Greer and figure out the cause of Kevin's issues and/or any treatment possible before we move on with trying to treat you."

I was fairly stunned at this news and not sure what to think of her use of the word "*problem.*" I mean, that stupid semen analysis was supposed to be *precautionary* she said, Just a *preventative* measure to ensure all was well. I was thinking, *What the heck do I do with all my plans?* I mentally, yet again, pushed aside my dreamed of due date and tried to reason out what to do next. As it was, I had very little time to process all this since I was to be picked up for the retreat in less than an hour. I proceeded to tell Kevin the news while choking back tears of my own, then went into my office, closed the door, called my mother, and utterly broke down. She tried to comfort me in her own way by warning me not to make *him* feel somehow like less of a man by being overly emotional myself (gee, thanks for that heaping side of guilt). Mom also told me not to panic until we saw Dr. Greer in the next week which was not, in and of itself, bad advice, but I was already two steps forward in my panic attack. Mom's sage advice fell on deaf ears.

I quickly ended that very unhelpful phone call and vowed to never go *first* to my mother for panic-stricken support. There was not even time to pray or talk to my husband about his feelings. I was still reeling a little from the news and not sure what to do with all my well-laid plans when I got a knock on my door and it was time to go to the retreat. And with that, I mustered all the courage I could find, sucked it up, put on a smile, grabbed my bags, and headed out the door.

Reeling

The drive up to the retreat with three other ladies in the car was pretty pleasant, all things considered. Everyone was chatting and making conversation, and really only my friend Jenny had any clue that not all was well in the Nelson household. I was cordial and even funny at times, and held together quite well, considering.

We got to the retreat and our rooms were fitted with little gift bags, goodies, and promises for good fun. I took a deep breath and thought, *this should be good for me. It will give me some time to process all this new information, and maybe get some good advice from other ladies. I could come home from this weekend rejuvenated, refreshed, and ready to overcome this tiny obstacle to my plans.* About here is where I realized God definitely does have a sense of humor and impeccable timing when I saw the theme for the retreat. "Bear One Another's Burdens." Or as I like to call it: the symphony of pain. And in case there was any doubt as to this weekend's intentions, the goodie bags even had a pack of tissues in them—I should have figured it out sooner that they intended this to be a tear-filled weekend. For me, it was a two day sob fest where we vacillated between super fun games filled with laughter and bonding, to benign crafts and workshops. Now, it is worth mentioning that being overly emotional is physically exhausting to me. I always feel *emotionally* better afterward, but *physically* I get drained and it often takes me a day to recover my energy when I fully melt down. As much as a good cry can be cathartic at times, I intentionally try to avoid that if possible when in a more public setting. And I *certainly* did *not* want to be a weepy mess the entire weekend at the retreat and let all of these women know what was going on in my bedroom. God has a wicked good sense of humor. Our first full day there was Saturday and we broke into groups of four to share our burdens and pray for each other. I quickly calculated that, with our time limit, I could volunteer to go last and then be skipped altogether when we ran out of time. I felt incredibly smart! Then I could take part in listening and sharing and bonding with everyone else, but not actually have to put myself "out there" for the world. Alas, no. The other women breezed through their life struggles in perfect form with five or less completed, coherent sentences, and then they all looked at me with anticipation. I feel confident that, at that moment, had a hole opened in the earth for me to jump into, I would have gladly leapt to my doom to avoid what I *knew* would be an emotional renting of my heart. Do not get me wrong, these women were *great* Christian women and were wonderfully supportive and caring to each other. But all their supportive and loving looks ripped off the very *thinly* veiled feeling of control I was holding onto and I felt completely—for lack of a better word—*naked*!

I tried to vaguely describe our conception difficulties in two or less succinct sentences, but what came out was a good five minute ramble amidst tears and that thing that happens to my voice where I try not to cry but then end up cry-talking at a pitch only dogs can hear. I avoided the details, at least I think I did, and summarized that we had started trying for a family and knew we had struggles on my side of the equation, but now found out that we have some unknown "problem" on Kevin's side too, and I was terrified that we would not be able to conceive at all. I also shared that this was all about twelve hours old and I had not had a chance to process it yet, and I think I even apologized for my basket case state. I pretty much rambled incoherently in a language that only other women who have been incoherent at some point in their lives could understand. These women were great—perfect, in fact—telling me not to be sorry for being emotional and then promptly praying for me and asking God to give me answers, grace, strength, etc. I personally prayed for strength, understanding, and for God to get us through this quickly and bring us *our* baby.

All the well wishes and kind words were a kind gesture on their part and, in truth, about the only thing they could have done, considering our time was now up and the whole group of nearly twenty-five women got together for more group games, laughing, and bonding. Anyone for an emotional sling shot?

The next day, we decided to walk into town for some retail therapy, which I adore and was glad for. I had slept well that night, woke up recharged, and was now shopping…things could not get much better than that. I felt confident I had passed the worst of the weekend's emotional roller coaster and would enjoy the rest of the day with the ladies. Again, God had other plans for me.

With the afternoon came another small group session to share burdens and pray for one another. Despite my failure at the last session's attempt to avoid this, I felt confident I could get out of this one. I had this plan that it would be the same three women with me and I would breeze past it with no explanation needed, and they would intuitively understand my desire to not share anymore at that point in time. I was so smart! I gave myself a mental gold star for my stellar plan and almost smugly thought, "Ha ha…you won't suck me in again!" But no, we numbered off and got into entirely new groups of four to share and bond with *other* women.

I immediately started calculating the ways I could gracefully squirm out of this. I was mortified at my own selfishness when I learned that someone else in my group had a serious concern of their own. As we listened to the other woman's concerns and offered our moral support, I was counting down the time. She talked and cried and we prayed for her, but even with all that, there were three minutes left. They all lovingly and supportively looked at me with those big puppy dog eyes, waiting for me to spill the beans. Really, where are those big "swallow you up" holes in the earth when you need them? Again, despite all my efforts at a more graceful display; I was sobbing while making futile attempts to contain myself. We then closed with more prayer and after that, it was group time.

When the weekend was finally over and we were all driving back home, I was not rejuvenated, or ready to attack and overcome this problem. I was exhausted, confused, guilt-ridden for my horrible thoughts and behavior. Only now, I was fairly sure I would not be "alone" in my prayers. A solid eight women at my church *knew* some far more private details of my life than I originally planned, and I could have won good money betting that even more women would know before the week was over. I could not see it at the time, but that weekend proved a brief glimpse, and a training ground, for the coming two years of my life. Exhaustive attempts at outward "normalcy," picking and choosing who you can and cannot share parts of your struggle with. A mix of seemingly futile prayers, emotional strains, and jarring moments that you must put on a smiling face and go on with the show, as they say. All the while having my own mind utterly filled with a slew of horrible obsessions on the extreme possibilities.

Even after that weekend, no one could have told me what I was in for and I was saturated with panic over the hurdles ahead of us. Still, each night, I would lay my head on my pillow and pray to God to bring us *our* baby. Deep down inside under the trepidation, I felt confident that we could overcome this and somehow all would be well. After all, we *had* only been trying six months now.

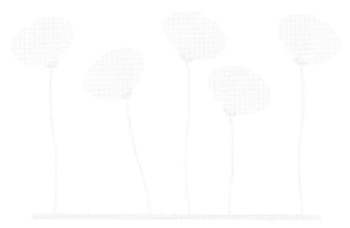

Bad to Worse to...
Wait a Second!

It was early May in 2007 when we drove to Dr. Greer's office, very unsure of what to expect. After all, from my limited female perspective, the urologist is like the male version of a gynecologist. I was expecting similar types of exams including, sadistically, the evil speculum and the need to "scoot to the end of the table."

We arrived, signed in, and proceeded to wait. Now—confirming my previous suspicions—there were anatomy pictures on the walls, but instead of female reproductive organs, it was all male. Weird cross sections of the male "piece" shown with little lines pointing out what everything is. I was slightly fascinated and a little oogged-out, which is, I would guess, what my husband feels at my doctor appointments. Dr. Greer came in and reintroduced himself and proceeded to go over the actual test results in detail. Truth be told, when we first found out that there were male factor issues by Dr. Hayes, I did not fully understand, or retain, much of what she said, as my brain fogged out a bit. Dr. Greer was surprisingly educational and made things seem a lot better than I had originally thought.

The end result was simply that my darling husband had such an overabundance of swimmers that the bad ones clumped up the good ones and the good ones never made it to their target destination. On the surface, that sounded good and I have to admit to puffing up my chest a bit because my man had an epic number of swimmers. I also began to feel slightly less panicky.

The good doctor went on to explain, in detail, the various tests they needed to run to try and find out the cause of the bad swimmers. It all seemed relatively benign and harmless. As we sat and listened to Dr. Greer rattle on about the antibody test, physical exam, blood work, repeat analysis, etc., I began to think that things might not be that bad and I slowly started to revisit my dream due dates and original plans. Then, for some crazy reason, I decided to ask, "Does this mean we can still move forward and try to conceive on our own with me taking the Clomid as Dr. Hayes had originally prescribed?"

He hesitated.

That is never a good sign.

Dr. Greer went on to tell us that we certainly can if we would like to, but our chances would be better if we did IUI.

Not Quite What We Had in Mind

As Dr. Greer explained, IUI is short for Intrauterine Insemination. The process involves me taking the Clomid, as planned, and tracking with ovulation predictor kits for my optimum days for "fun." However, instead of actually having "the fun," we would call his office and rush a sample of Kevin's swimmers in for washing by a lab. The washing procedure would remove the bad swimmers and hype up the good swimmers in special fluid that gave them more energy. I envisioned this to be the Red Bull for sperm. Then, Dr. Greer would insert a catheter through my cervix into my uterus and inject only the good swimmers, thus giving my husband's boys the best possible head start. Needless to say, that last part was not planned, but it all sounded good on paper. Sadly, my vision of the two of us conceiving in an act of marital passion and memorable perfection was cracked and flawed forever at this point. I tried to reconcile in my mind that one day our darling child would ask where babies come from and I would have to answer, "Well, mommy and daddy fell in love and got married. Then we saw a slew of medical specialists and they decided how best to help Mr. Stork find us."

I stared off into nothing and mentally buried my hopes for a natural conception. It was a beautiful funeral. As my imaginary memorial ended, my ever practical husband looked at Dr. Greer and asked, "What are our chances if we do this IUI," to which Dr. Greer dutifully rattled off the standard stats. The ones that say even the healthiest, normal couple has about a 20 percent chance per cycle to conceive, and that with IUI, our odds would be around 10 percent or better. This was not a great number, but not horrible, and in my mind I was still relatively holding on to hope that we would come out of this and be "okay." Then, my darling, lovable, ever cost-effective husband asked about the financial outgo of all this. Truly it was and is his nature, he could not help himself. We were told it would run us about $350.00–500.00 per cycle and could take three to six cycles for success. We thought that sounded like a lot of money for only a 10 percent chance, but what choice did we have? My next question was, "What are the odds if we just try on our own to conceive with the Clomid, insuring ovulation, but avoiding IUI costs and trying the natural method?"

Dr. Greer hesitated.

Again. I quickly learned to hate hesitation in the medical profession.

He then said, "Given your anovulatory cycles, and with your husband's current sperm analysis numbers… even with Clomid you have roughly 5 to 7 percent chance *at best*."

Hold The Phone!

I was just told that my husband has an astronomical amount of swimmers. In my mind, less is not more… *more is more… bigger is better!* How could his overabundance of swimmers somehow lessen our chances? Questions raced through my mind as an anvil dropped on my brain. Dr. Greer went on to explain that antioxidants can help Kevin's numbers a little, but it takes three months or more to see any result, and yes, we can try for a few months if we want and then come back for IUI blah blah blah. At that point, all I heard was, "Ma'am, you have a snowball's chance in hell of conceiving on your own. Kiss those dreamed of due dates good-bye and get ready for expensive IUI cycles."

The drive home from that appointment was agony. It was the normal twenty-minute drive really, but now seemed deafening. You know those kinds of drives where the conversation is thunderous *in your head* but the car is full of awkward silence. I knew that my darling husband wanted to try the natural way…because it was *cheaper*. I knew he would want to put our family plans on hold to save a buck. My mind was gearing up for a good battle. I was lining up my argument to get my way and trying to pad myself for whatever he might say to refute what I wanted.

I sat in the car desperately wanting to schedule our first IUI as soon as possible to continue moving forward *quickly*. I had an overwhelming fear that we would never have success unless we acted immediately, and without Dr. Greer and the IUI team, we would no doubt be childless forever! I knew that if we did not hurry our chances would slip away. And to top off all the noise in my head, the guilt of my past indiscretions slipped into an unbearable feeling that I somehow deserved this. I was slowly starting to think that my former life—my life before Kevin and before my solid relationship with Christ. My very skewed and sin-filled, misguided life—was the cause of all this. I prayed silently that this was not the case, but at that time, the only thing in my mind was—I had this coming.

We drove on and as my mind lined up the firing squad ready to shoot down any ideas that came my way, Kevin verbalized his desire to try antioxidants, vitamins, and Clomid. He wanted to try on our own for three months, and see what happened.

It is worth noting at this point that my husband has always had massive amounts of faith that all will be fine. This little hiccup in our family planning efforts was just that to him, a little hiccup. We would overcome this. There was no doubt in his mind, and after all, we had only been at it for seven months now.

We could not afford IUI in the immediate future, he reasoned, and waiting would let us save up a bit and not go into more debt. He also felt confident it would work and we would conceive on our own in no time at all and not even need IUIs. I said nothing and mentally began loading my shotgun with rebuttals.

I started feeling more and more suffocated by my own lack of verbalization while he continued to justify his thoughts to me. I wanted to scream at my husband that I could not stand to wait that long and I wanted a baby *now*. Now, now, *now*! I wanted to tell him how scared I was that we'd loose precious time on nothing, and I wanted to remind him that while he's taking those multivitamins for three months and breezing through this time period, I will be hopped up on Clomid, and that it was not fair of him to be choosing this route on his own without considering the toll it would take on *me*.

Meanwhile, over the noise of all those things I wanted to say, there was still a small voice in the back of my mind that said, *Now honey, the more natural way might work. Antioxidants are cheaper than IUI, and you do not need more debt in your life right now with all the debt you already have. And sweetie, you need to respect the fact that your husband is not ready for IUI yet and he needs some time to come to grips with all this too. This is not only about you, but both of you as a couple, and the choice should be made together… not you stamping your foot like a spoiled child and demandin' your way.*

In the end, despite all the vapid ranting that was inside my head, all the perfectly stated arguments lined up and ready to go, I begrudgingly agreed to Kevin's decision. We decided to purchase vitamin supplements, more organic fruits and veggies and juices to boost Kevin's immune system, and I would do Clomid. We would try on our own for a few months. I guess I could not disagree too much. We *were* heavily in debt at this point, and each month was slightly stressful to get all the bills paid and have anything left over for fun, much less savings and extra medical costs. It was, in the end, the smarter and more mature route to go, I guess. But I did *not* like it one itty bitty bit.

Compromise and Moving Forward

After telling Dr. Hayes of our plans, she agreed and called in my Clomid prescription (50mg per day). She instructed me to take it on cycle days five through nine, and then start tracking my ovulation to find the optimum "sheet frolicking" time. So, as instructed, when my period started that June 2007 I counted until cycle day five and started the Clomid. Here is a rough emotional assessment of the days that followed:

- Day five: feeling fine with no noticeable side effects.
- Day six: feeling fine but nervous and a little edgy.
- Day seven: starting to feel a little jumpy and irritable.
- Day eight: short fused and easily lit.
- Day nine: DEFCON 1, flash fire temper, keep a safe distance.

I really thought that the first three days were a breeze and those women who complained about Clomid were a little overly dramatic. I had done my research on the drug and lots of women complained of hot flashes and mood swings and such, but I thought I was having an easy time of it at first. *This is a breeze,* I thought. Of course, I also thought to myself that perhaps this was a sign it was not working, which is perfect for my nature to find something reassuring and immediately follow it up with a worry of some kind. So with every day I took my pills, I prayed silently that God would make them work and be *super* effective and give us *our* baby.

Any fears I had of the Clomid not being effective were laid to rest on day eight. I remember that day vividly because I had to go grocery shopping and I ran into a lovely older woman that we used to go to church with. She was great, but notoriously chatty with just about anyone and everyone. I was already feeling a bit wound up because of the teaming hordes of grocery shoppers that had barred my path to the toilet paper and caused a near emotional meltdown over the paper towel selection. When the lovely, let's call her Ms. Chatty, decided to stop my cart and catch me up on her entire life story in aisle six, it was about all I could do to contain myself. I feel confident that if a psychologist had read my mind at that moment I would have sounded perfectly schizophrenic. One part of me was saying to be calm and remember that this old woman likely did not have a lot of people to talk to. She was very sweet, and why was I in such a hurry anyway? The other part of me was seriously contemplating some fake emergency so I could run away from the grocery store as fast as possible. I was mentally tallying how rude and arrogant this old bag was for holding me up on such an important errand to get milk. Yet, another part of me was still silently praying for composure and grace under the great emotional strain of the day that had overtaxed me. Of course, all of this was under the surface of a perfectly calm face and polite conversation that not one soul realized was a *façade*.

By the time I finally got into my car, passive-aggressively slamming every door I could safely slam in the process, I was thoroughly steaming mad. In fact, I spent the entire drive home further reviewing the inter-action and building up the "case" in my mind even further.

By the time I got home I was fuming angry. As Kevin helped me unload the groceries he calmly asked, "What's wrong" after I *subtly* sighed, slammed, grumbled, and huffed my way through the house. I proceeded to relay the whole trip to him (while slamming groceries into their appropriate locations). I ended my rant with a statement that Ms. Chatty was a fat old windbag that did not know when to shut her pie-hole, and she held up my grocery trip by nearly ten minutes blabbering on about totally unimportant crap! I even shared with him my experi-ence with the crazy nut jobs at the grocery store who did not know basic shopping cart etiquette enough to stay on the *right side* of the freaking aisle…and how much time did you need to stand and stare at toilet paper anyway? Why could not they all get the heck out of my way?

Kevin stood there—jaw firmly on the floor—shocked. When I finally took a breath from my semi-rehearsed rant, he laughed a little and said he'd never heard me speak that way of Ms. Chatty, or anyone else for that matter. I sort of laughed a little too and said, "I know, I do not know what came over me, she just drove me nuts." Kevin then decided, in his sick sense of humor, to list off a few names of other people we know to see my response and sure enough, everyone he listed was on my hit list for some reason or another, and I was able to instantly spew out some awful description of their perceived flaw, thus confirming how awful I was and exactly how much Clomid *was* taking its toll on me. Thankfully, he stopped before asking me about my mother or his mother or *anyone's* mother, because who knows what I would have said. We then realized that Clomid was indeed working and we had a good laugh about the whole ordeal. At that moment, however, I made a little mental note to start being more aware of my thoughts. Clomid or not, I thought to myself, I could *not* let this ruin relationships with friends and family members. Clomid or no, I would *not* lose myself to this kind of bitter existence.

The Importance of Laughter

The next day, the final dose of Clomid was taken and I resigned to stay in the house if I could. I was anxious and edgy, but otherwise holding my own okay; I would not subject the world at-large to my very sensitive emotional state.

Lunchtime rolled around and we met in the kitchen as usual to fix sandwiches, etc. I stood at the stove doing something (I do not know what) and my husband opened the microwave to pull out his lunch. As he did, he failed to completely close the microwave door and it slowly crept back open. Now, by slowly, I mean *snail's pace* slowly, and even a toddler could have seen, registered, and ducked out of the way of the oncoming door. Nonetheless, I did *not* notice it or register that it was swinging open, despite Kevin's warning of, "Watch your head." About that time, I looked up, the door ever so lightly tapped me on the forehead and immediately *the gloves came off!* I explosively slammed the door of the microwave so hard that and it literally whistled as it flew by. Kevin barely got his hand out of the way before there were broken fingers involved. I widened my stance, gripped my knife in my hands with white-knuckle intensity, and in total seriousness, growled *"Bring it on!"* To the microwave! At that moment, I was plotting the death of the vile microwave and all kitchen appliances that opposed me. *Death to the blender!* Kevin stood there with this amused but shocked look on his face as he watched me transform from his normally loving wife to a WWF wrestler in mere seconds, and then again transform back, as the hackles smoothed down and I released the knife in my hand.

Then—and only then—he did it. I do not know how or why or even how he knew it was safe to do—but he did it. He broke into hysterical belly-filling laughter. Most men at this point would have, intelligently, run for the nearest man cave so as to not incur the wrath of a hormonal nut job. Not my sweetie. He laughed till his belly jiggled and tears misted the corners of his eyes. He laughed so hard and with so much pure joy in his eyes that I laughed too. He said he could not believe what I was doing and that it was very unlike me and he felt *bad* for me for having to go through all that, but that it was uproariously funny.

In that instant, I loved him a little more. Not for laughing *at* me, but for laughing at the situation and loving me and not judging my completely insane reactions. What a wondrous gift God had given me. God knew that one day in our marriage I would need an unreasonable amount of understanding, He divinely gave me a husband with patience in abundance. What a *great* God!

Kevin and I laughed together and I felt much better. We both chalked it up to that last dose of Clomid and went about our day. Inside, I was grateful and thanked God for giving me a husband that was willing to love me despite my flaws, and could help me find humor and not take myself so dang seriously… even during a serious time.

The rest of June was relatively uneventful. We had somewhat informed family of our plans, but not really gone into detail. I ovulated on the Clomid and we "did the deed" and waited the appropriate two weeks. Once the appropriate time arrived, we took a home pregnancy test (HPT) and it came up quickly and firmly negative. We waited for my cycle to start and try again. In the meantime, we were saving up every penny we could for future IUI cycles. However, a family trip to the South to visit my father and stepmother was planned. Even though we could have afforded the IUI, we would be gone. About that time, our only car was in dire need of brakes, and guess how much it cost. The cost to fix the brakes is exactly how much we had saved up in cash, almost to the penny. Since we could not do the IUI because of travel anyway, that money was used to put new brakes on our only vehicle. Coincidence… I think not!

In early July, my period started again, and again Dr. Hayes called me in another perscription of Clomid. We had been trying to conceive for a total of nine solid months with now two months of Clomid to assist us. I took this time to finally inform my family of our situation, in more detail, and to ask for prayer and support. I had pseudo-clued them in that we were having struggles. It was easy since like most good Southern families, by telling the key people, everyone pretty much knew what was going on. I decided e-mail was the easiest way to communicate. It was on my terms, sharing only what I wanted to share, and avoided me having to make phone call after phone call to Alabama, Mississippi, Texas, Washington, etc., to repeat the gritty details over and over again. My e-mail went something like this:

Hey guys, I have not sent out an update since the end of May-ish, so I figured now was as good a time as any.

You all know that the Clomid worked, which is great. But, we're still trying. We are starting round two of Clomid today. We feel confident it will work again, which is good. However, the timing may not be great. We are flying out of Boise to visit Dad on the 30th. Depending on when the Clomid kicks in, our "optimum time" to have a trip to the doctor for IUI will likely be while we are in, Mississippi. Really, that just means we will postpone our first IUI cycle again until the next month. Our chances without it are around 5 to 10 ten percent, so it's not likely we'll be successful on our own… but who knows.

Anyway, that's the plan. On a semi-related note, our first shot to do IUI, we did not have the cash, but we've been saving. Now we are ready, but will be out of town. Oddly, now was the time we needed to get our car fixed (needed brakes) and it cost just under what we had saved, so timing wise, it was perfect for us to be able to pay cash for that and still have time to save up again for when we are back in town. I guess God is planning this for us and we can hang around for the ride.

PS: Keep praying for us. This is not really exciting news yet, but frankly it ain't a baby yet either so do not stop the prayers and good vibes.

My family responded with the usual platitudes and good wishes and benign questions, but mostly kept silent and waited, like us.

The second month of Clomid was as trying for me, but I had learned my lesson and we pretty much stayed home as much as possible, which helped keep the outward forces of frustration away from me. We did have a funny moment involving a milk carton and my anger at the dairy association for making them square, but that is a less funny story than the microwave one so I'll skip it for now.

After we finished that Clomid round and started tracking ovulation, we also packed our bags for a five-day vacation in Mississippi at my dad's house. All my brothers and their families would be there for the Fourth of July and, living in Idaho as we did, we did not get to see them much. I was excited to go. Being that the timing was close, we packed along our special baby-making lubricant that we had ordered online, and the ovulation predictor kits so we could make sure and not miss our optimal time. I was not sure how all that would work at my father's house, but we were determined to try our best.

Sure enough, that test lit up right on July 3 and we did the deed on July 4 as instructed. Granted it was not fireworks and romance since we were at my dad's house after all. We were not going to let that slow us down, though. In fact, as we laid there, with me propped up on pillows and such, my husband and I actually talked about how cool it would be if this baby was conceived *on* July 4 of all days, and how neat of a story it would be, and how excited my Dad would be that it happened at his house, etc. Part of me even mentally revisited my baby dreams and had a small modicum of hope. I prayed hard that God would let all these things be and that He would bless us with *our* baby.

When the trip was over, we flew back home and proceeded to wait the full amount of time before taking a home pregnancy test. Technically, I was supposed to take it on a Friday, but starting about Tuesday/Wednesday I was not feeling like myself. My boobs were sore, and my normally legendary appetite was nonexistent When my husband realized Wednesday night that I had not touched my dinner, he insisted I take a pregnancy test right at that moment. We happened to have a few tests layring around so I pee'd on the stick and low-and-behold—a faint second line. Granted it was a few days early, and it was nighttime rather than the optimum morning requirement, but it was definitely there. I was not sure I was seeing it and my husband double-checked and agreed…that beautiful, gorgeous, perfect in every way test said we were definitely, totally, completely pregnant!

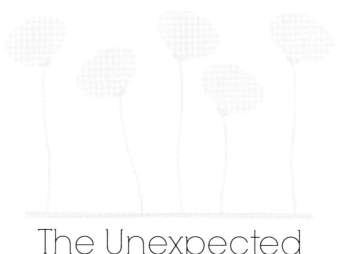

The Unexpected

Discovering that the little pee stick said "pregnant" was a shock, to say the least. My husband immediately ran out and bought me more tests. They had to be digital this time so we could be sure. While he was at the store, he also grabbed celebratory pickles and ice cream too. I tested again and sure enough… pregnant. We then proceeded to call our parents and close friends and shout the news to all who could hear. My dad was expectantly proud that we had actually conceived in Mississippi, and our friends who had prayed for us were elated. We were thrilled and had an abundance of people praying for us already. It was such a shock to take it all in. Here we were earmarking funds for IUI next month and instead we get this unexpected plus sign; we couldn't shout the news loud enough to say the least.

To be extra *double* for sure, first thing the next morning I tested one more time and sure enough, I was still pregnant. I called Dr. Hayes and we made an appointment for my first OB checkup and sonogram in the coming weeks. I smiled from ear to ear when the nurse asked me what type of appointment I needed and I got to tell *her* the good news too. Our prayers had been answered and we were expecting our first child. Cloud *Ten* is a good description of where we were. My husband strutted around with well-earned pride. Not only did "his boys" do the job on their own without IUI's, but his faith had proven steadfast. I was reveling in my new pregnant state. I loved each and every "how are you feeling" and "I heard the good news" that I got at church. I was not nauseated, per se, but did have other symptoms to go along with the pregnancy, like sore boobs, aching back, and a freakish craving for vinegary foods. I enjoyed every pain, every twinge, and every ounce of discomfort I had. I was a pregnant, soon-to-be mother and nothing compared. We prayed and thanked God each night for our baby and asked that He keep both of us healthy and strong for the coming months.

We were thrilled at our first doctor's appointment. First, was the usual first time pregnant parent's Q&A with Dr. Hayes. She was fantastic and addressed any and all questions we both had. Then was the blessed ultrasound which, invasive as it was, allowed us to see our little baby. He was beautiful, measuring right at seven weeks three days and a heartbeat that was fast and strong. I was mesmerized, as was Kevin. What more could expectant parents ask for than a black and white dot with a flickering heartbeat? We were instantly in love with our little peanut shaped blob and in fact, that is what we named the baby. From then on, it was not "the baby" or "it"… it was Peanut—our first child. We would forever introduce our baby's sonogram photo to others by asking if they wanted to meet our Peanut. Finally, my dreams of our future family were in full swing.

Our estimated due date was March 24, 2008. Kevin was practically giggly at that since it was the day after his birthday. We were both a little shocked at how far along we were. We figured I was about two or three weeks pregnant. However, that new fangled "period math" is done a bit differently and we were twice that far into things. We were nearly eight weeks pregnant already. I was shocked that we got to actually *see* the baby's heartbeat and Kevin was kicking himself for not having the ability to somehow record the momentous occasion. Our beautiful baby's movement was not only a surprise to us, but marked that we were already over halfway through the first trimester. Being unprepared like that was simply unacceptable now that we were parent's. We immediately left the doctor's office with our next appointment schedule for four weeks away and some instructions on do's and don'ts of pregnancy. As we walked to the car, Kevin announced that we needed to make a quick trip to the local electronics store to purchase a digital camera and camcorder so that at the next appointment, we would be ready. He even bought the camcorder accessories, a digital camera for me, and a special backpack to hold it all. He named the backpack, "The Dad-Bag." We both dreamed big and were grateful to finally be in the special club we so longed for; Parenthood.

Those next four weeks crept by for us. We continued our life as normal, working and attending/volunteering at church in our various ministries, etc. But inside, we were biding our time until our next appointment, which would mark the second trimester and a new look at the bigger, better, and stronger Peanut. We bought pregnancy books and read them fervently. My husband's personal favorite was "Girlfriends Guide to Pregnancy," which he laughed all the way through. I liked the practical and comical insight from that book, but loved the pregnancy guide by the Mayo Clinic that showed what our baby looked like each week and gave us a practical size comparison. It was fun to envision our baby and wonder how it looked.

Our families also got into the enthusiasm. We immediately got flowers from family and gifts from friends. My family down in Dallas sent some new baby things, as well as a new purse and jewelry for mom-to-be. After all, celebratory occasions of any kind require a new purse! My dad in Mississippi took personal pride in the fact that Peanut was derived on his home turf, and said it was a sign that we should then move to Mississippi for all future family rearing.

Friends locally got into the action too, giving us small gifts and asking for all the news. Of course who could blame them. By then, we had nearly half the church praying for us and our struggles. It was understandable that they would all now be equally thrilled to see those prayers answered quickly and completely. Each Sunday at church was marked by how many people would come up and ask us how Peanut was doing and when Peanut's due date was. As a parent, I felt a certain pride that everyone had jumped on board the fact that our baby was "named" Peanut, and that this pregnancy was a blessing to others, as well as myself. Probably my favorite though, we had some friends of ours who were also expecting, and their due date was nearly identical to ours. Each Sunday the other mom and I would get to compare pregnancy notes on our respective weight gain, clothing issues, doctor's appointments, etc.

From the perspective of an expectant mother, life could not have gotten any better than that moment. To go from such sadness and fear to such happiness almost overnight, and then to have that joy shared and reverberated by so many others, was euphoric.

Toward the end of the first trimester I started noticing that my pregnancy symptoms had all but stopped. My back/tailbone still hurt, but my boobs felt normal and my appetite was back on track. Deep down, in the dark recesses of my mind where I manufacture worries on a day-to-day basis, I wondered if this was a bad sign that something was not quite right. I mentioned it to my stepmother and my husband, both of whom said I was worrying needlessly. They agreed that it was likely a sign that we were getting into that second trimester bliss—the holy land of pregnancy, if you will—where things start feeling better. In truth, I was reading one of the scariest pregnancy books on the market and had a tendency to worry anyway. It made sense that I was building this up in my mind as I often tended to do. I tried to put the worries out of my mind; I hid that stupid book and looked forward to my next appointment.

When that glorious Thursday in September 2007 arrived, we showed up, enthusiastically early, to Dr. Hayes's office with camcorder and goofy grins in tow. I even remember that the song "Praise You in This Storm" by Casting Crowns was playing, and we both commented to each other about how much we liked the lyrics. I remember thinking, we'll never hear this song again that we do not think of this wonderful day that all our worries and fears were unfounded and our prayers were answered, and God had a plan and had, in fact, carried us through this rough patch. I remember too, I even giggled like a school girl while reading the pregnancy magazines in the waiting room, after all, these were for me now.

This was an easier appointment in that I did not have to totally strip, but rather had a quick chat with the Dr. Hayes and a Doppler check for Peanut's heartbeat. We were told that we would not have an ultrasound until twenty weeks, which we were bummed about, but what could we do. I laid back, Dr. Hayes gooped up my belly, and we all held our breath and waited to hear the heartbeat. We could not find it at first and Dr. Hayes said that it was still early, and that it's sometimes hard to find the heartbeat each time. She told us not to be concerned. We all waited some more as Dr. Hayes' eyes went off to a distant stare, and she concentrated and moved the Doppler around on my belly. We waited, and waited, and waited some more. Dr. Hayes then stated that she was not hearing what she wanted to hear, but that could mean that the baby was curled up and hiding. She offered to give us an ultrasound to ease everyone's mind. Kevin and I both smiled and nearly high-fived. He would finally get to use his camcorder, and I specifically recall looking down at my belly and saying, "Way to go, Peanut… way to get another picture for mommy… good job!"

I was practically skipping into the ultrasound room and I'm pretty sure I leapt back into the stirrups. Dr. Hayes again stated that this early, sometimes you cannot find the heartbeat with the Doppler and this ultrasound would quickly confirm that all was well. She gingerly inserted the probe and dimmed the lights and we waited, and waited, and waited some more. Just as I was about to worry, I looked up and saw our little Peanut on the screen. My heart went all gooey as I gazed at my gorgeous Peanut-shaped blob… but Dr. Hayes, however, was silent. Her eyes were again in a distant, concentrated stare as she moved the probe around and watched the baby closely. She kept looking around on the sonogram machine, and then said the most gut-wrenching words I had ever heard in my entire life up to that point. "I'm sorry guys, but it looks like we've lost him."

Ton of Bricks

Nothing in the history of the world could have prepared me for that moment. I felt the air leave my lungs, as if Dr. Hayes had physically punched me in the gut. I wanted to yell "*What do you mean we lost him? Is he still in there and hiding? Check again!*" But we stared at the screen, dumbfounded. Sure enough, our little baby was there. I could see Peanut—our little gray blob—on the screen, as we had seen before, only, no flicker. If possible, my mind had gone simultaneously into overdrive of questions and completely numb of emotion, which left me plain speechless in the torrent. Dr. Hayes softly pointed out that Peanut was still inside me, but only measuring about eight weeks and had no heartbeat. At thirteen weeks, Peanut should have been much larger, with a strong heartbeat and visible arms and legs and that precious movement we hoped to see. It appeared Peanut had been gone for quite some time now and my ignorant, horrible, broken, defunct body did not catch on. I looked at my husband half expecting to see anger in his face, but he too stared at the screen, totally silent.

It is amazing how vivid the memory of these times can be. I sat up on the table, still draped in paper from the waist down, and asked numbly, "Well, what now?" Dr. Hayes laid out the options very simply for us. She gave us three options to choose from basically:

- "I'm willing to let you wait up to another four weeks for your body to take care of this on its own, naturally."

- "There is some medication we can give you to take at home to help start the process and then let you naturally complete the process from there."

- "We can schedule a D & C and go in and remove things here in the office."

Dr. Hayes made it very clear that the choice was completely ours and we could take a day or two to think it over if needed. She would support us either way. My mind marveled at her use of the words "its" and "the process" and "things." In the short few minutes we were in that horrible shrinking room, Peanut had been reduced from a baby with a heartbeat and a future—to an "its." I was angry for Peanut. I then asked the most horrid and masochistic question that I could think of. I said, "A few weeks back, I noticed my pregnancy symptoms had decreased dramatically and I was worried that there was something wrong, but I figured it was second trimester stuff. Could this have been what I was feeling… that the baby was gone?" On the surface, this question seemed honest and harmless, but the answer had the potential to ruin me completely and it was only my own morbid sense of self-flagellation that made me ask. In reality, I was looking for the doctor to confirm that I should have done something sooner to prevent this, and in my failure, I was to blame for Peanut's death. Dr. Hayes, in her gentle way, answered, "Normally I would say that all was likely fine, but given what we know about the baby's size, it is possible that something else was going on. It is impossible to tell, at losses this early on, what the real cause could have been." My heart sank. I was right. Why did I not trust my instincts?

Even as the doctor explained repeatedly that these things happen, and she even rattled off statistics of how frequently these things happen, I knew that part of me had somehow caused this by not listening to my instincts. As a mother, I had already failed utterly and completely, and it cost my first child his life. Wolves would have done a better job at bringing Peanut into the world and raising him.

Dr. Hayes, likely sensing my inner panic, was very quick to reassure me that even had I rushed into the office that very day, there was nothing that could have been done because I was too early in the pregnancy. She tried to reassure me, over and over, that during the first trimester, nothing could have been done had we known the day *before* that something was going to happen much less the day of or after and that I did *nothing* wrong to cause this. I stared at her. I did not even cry. Honestly, I do not remember at all if Kevin said a single word at this point, as I was numb. I can remember the shirt I was wearing and the shoes the doctor had on, but I cannot remember if my husband said anything to me at that point.

As the doctor left the room, I got up and went to the bathroom to clean up and put my clothes back on. I sat on the toilet and when I stood up to put my shoes on; I glanced in the bowl and realized I was looking for blood. That was the straw that broke the camel's back, as they say. I was actually *looking* for signs of my dead baby to be vacating my body. The very thought made me abhor myself.

At that point, the tears started falling hard and fast. Or rather, the dam burst and the tears could not fall fast enough. I do not remember checking out of the doctor's office, but I remember failing miserably at my attempts to hold it together as we left the hospital and got to our car. I was drowning in the rushing waves of emotions. Fear that I had caused this, guilt that I did not stop this, pain and sadness and embarrassment and anger and horror... it all hit me within minutes.

The walk from the doctor's sonogram room to our car was the longest gauntlet of emotions I had ever experienced. It lasted forever, but I hardly remember the steps I took. I am sure we passed people, but could not tell you if they looked our way or politely turned their heads as the haze of my depression floated by.

I clearly remember that when we got in the car, Kevin finally broke down, which snapped me out of things a bit. Prior to this, the few tears I had seen him shed in the course of our entire relationship were mild, few, and far between. But this time, his expression shocked me. I had never seen this level of despair on his face. He got me in the car, walked around and put his dad-bag in the car, and closed the driver's side door. He sat there, sobbing. He looked as heartbroken and hopeless as I had ever seen him. Eyes and nose red, tears streaming, sobbing unlike anything I had ever seen in a man. It shocked me enough that my crying ceased, but I watched him. I ached to comfort him, but couldn't... I did not know how. I wanted him to know how much I loved him for being sad, but couldn't... I did not know how. I watched him as he cried and added his crushing despair to my own list of guilts. He commented that, "That was not just a baby... it was Peanut—*our* Peanut," a comment we later heard almost identically from my father-in-law. My heart broke a little bit more at hearing his attachment and sorrow, and I did not know how we would ever recover from this.

The drive home was a blur, with the exception that the song "Praise You in This Storm" by Casting Crowns was playing *again* on the radio and I remember thinking, we'll never hear this song again that we do not think of this awful, horrible, heartbreaking moment. We took back roads to avoid traffic and drove through a fast-food joint for dinner. Heck, we even rented movies and somehow ended up at home not quite sure what to do or say. I could not even tell you what movie we watched, and I do not think I ate two bites of food. We were both in shock from the afternoon and I wanted to crawl in a hole and hide forever. But one thing we did have to do was tell our families, and *that* was a task I did not think I could bear alone so we divvied up the responsibility.

I first called my mother. As soon as she answered and I said, "Mom," she knew. She immediately asked what was wrong and I all I could manage to say was, "We lost the baby." Indeed the tears were free-flowing at this point, and it was all I could do to answer what questions she had. The expected ones, "Do they know why" and "What happens now?" I did my best to explain the appointment with her and she agreed to tell my brothers, and aunts, and cousins for me. I was grateful to be spared that at least. I then called my stepmother, and that call was even harder. Not only was I crying and sobbing, but she was too. She was sorry and wished she could be in Idaho with us so we were not so alone. I found myself then worrying about *her* crying and feeling awful for having failed this pregnancy for the both of us. Mentally, I added that little emotion to my laundry list of reasons why I was a horrible mother.

My last call was to my friend at church who I asked the horrible favor of telling our other church friends. It was an awful bit of news to ask of anyone to share, and I was forever indebted to her for doing it. I made a point, somehow, to tell her to please tell our other pregnant friends to please *not* feel bad about talking to us and that we were still very happy for their pregnancy, but that was about all I could do at that point.

By the end of that phone call, I had run out of energy to maintain much more than my level of breathing. This left my husband with the task of telling his parents and sister, and I honestly do not know what he said or what they said. I was fully emotionally drained and drowning at the same time and could not have told you what day it was, much less keep track of anything else. The debilitating grief had finally won and it was all I could do to climb into bed. There were no prayers that night.

That night, sleep was solid from exhaustion, but blessedly dreamless. The next morning I woke up with the usual pregnancy sensations of having to pee and my back was hurting, and it shattered my heart into a million tiny pieces all over again. I realized, right then, I could not sit around and wait up to four weeks for this nightmare to happen. It felt too much like *waiting* for my baby to fall out of me. Furthermore, I could not go on *feeling* pregnant and knowing my baby was dead. Kevin supported whatever decision I wanted, but he was leaning to avoid a D & C if possible. We both agreed that felt too much like an abortion and we opted for the medication to get things going. I called the doctor, and she personally called me back and phoned in the prescription, along with detailed instructions of when to take it and what to expect, physically. She was professional and thorough but in the end, she was very soft and kind and non-judgmental, which I appreciated greatly. If you could have looked at the floor of my life at that moment, you would have seen the tiniest of shards of my broken heart all around me. The pieces of my life were in fragments and I did not see how I would ever put them back to whole the way they were.

It was amazing to me how other people reacted to our situation. Our boss (we both worked from home for the same company) gave us the day off and any other time we needed. I suppose he had little choice, considering his lead programmer and only sales rep were both a wreck and could not have functioned to save our lives. Aside from his understanding tone, our boss had little else to say by words of comfort or encouragement, but what could we have expected anyway from a newlywed guy with no kids of his own?

HEATHER D. NELSON

We immediately started getting cards and phone calls and e-mails from family and friends expressing concern as well. We asked for some privacy during the following few days and for the most part, everyone respected that. I did have an increase in phone calls from women who had experienced miscarriages themselves. They were eager to express their concern, share their experiences, and let me know they were there. They were great—each and every one of them—but I was not ready to hear them yet.

Friday, the day after that horrible, fateful doctor visit, my husband asked me what I wanted to do, and I said I needed to get out of the house. I could not work, but could not sit around staring at the walls waiting for the prescription either. He was an angel, and we decided to go have dinner and see a movie and get out of the house. Dinner was not what I had in mind, but turned out to be good for me. He always knows what I need, even when I do not.

We ordered a bottle of my favorite wine and after having a glass, I was relaxed enough to actually *talk* a little bit without breaking down. It gave us a chance to hash out some things that needed discussing. He admitted that he got most of his crying out of the way the night before and was still sad, but was more concerned for me at this point. I admitted that I could not handle the guilt of walking around still feeling pregnant (back aches and needing to pee all the time), but knowing that my baby was dead. I also told him that I felt I needed to do something to honor this baby when the time came. I did not want to move on, try again, have a family, and ignore Peanut as if he meant nothing to us because he was not strong enough to make it full-term. He agreed with me fully on that point, and I was glad I put it out there and verbalized that. We discussed what I wanted to do and I had two main things in mind. One was a necklace to be made with Peanut's original birthstone on it, and the other was a small scrapbook album documenting the happiness that Peanut had brought us. Those were things I would have done anyway had Peanut been born into our lives, and I felt we owed it to him to continue with that plan. Kevin had something he wanted to do as well, but I do not honestly recall what it was.

On our way home, we picked up the medication and planned for a weekend "in" to get this part past us. At that point, I decided I was done crying. I wanted this over, and I cried no more. We even had a dear, wonderful friend bring over dinner for us and I did not even cry then. I did not pray, I did not cry, I was decidedly ready to get this over with and move on.

I took the medication as prescribed and was told that I should expect cramping and then heavy bleeding, etc. So we waited… and waited… and waited. The weekend was a blur of me living on the couch in my sweat-pants and running to the bathroom at every twinge "down there" to check for blood. It was awful. *I* was awful. I supposedly wanted this baby so very badly, but now I wanted this to be over with. I felt like I was *wishing* for the bleeding to start. *No wonder,* I thought to myself, *Why would God give me a baby when I'm wishing it away so quickly.* You'd think I would have relished the feeling of being pregnant a little longer and longed to hold on to Peanut as long as I could. Instead, I wanted Peanut out of me and I wanted completion. That was one more heaping side dish of guilt I added to my mental list of why I was a horrible mother.

Alas, the weekend came and went, and nothing happened. Not a cramp, not a drop of blood, nothing. Monday, I called Dr. Hayes. It was her day off, but she graciously called me back personally and even gave me her home phone if I needed it. I explained that nothing happened with the medication, and she explained that we were back at square one and she was willing to give us all three of the original options again. I asked her if a second round of that medication would work, to which she replied, "Well, we would have thought the first round would have worked, it's hard to say." I laughed to myself and thought, *Well, ya* can't *knock an honest answer now can ya?* I could not see repeating something that already failed and the waiting around for a month was too much. I finally confessed to Kevin that I could not do this anymore. Walking around like a zombie and waiting for my baby to fall out of me was too much to bear, and I desperately needed this to be over. The good doctor said she understood and Kevin agreed as well, and we scheduled the D & C for later that week.

At this point, after my family being told and the pastor announcing our loss to the church congregation, we were getting a flood of cards and calls that were all largely ignored. Nonetheless, I figured an update was in order, but I could not stand the thought of all those phone calls and questions. As tacky as I knew it was, I decided that an email was the next best thing.

> Okay, e-mail is way impersonal for something like this, but it's too hard to call everyone, and I'm forgetting who knows what and who does not know, so I figured one message now would not hurt. Just to catch anyone up on what's happened until now. We went in last Thursday for a regular checkup and found out there was no heartbeat and the baby was gone. We also found out that the baby had been gone for three-plus weeks.
>
> We were told we had three options:
>
> • Wait up to another month for my body to figure out what to do on its own.
>
> • Take a prescription to kick-start the process.
>
> • D & C (an office procedure to take care of things quickly/ completely/medically).
>
> We opted for medication—did that over the weekend—nothing happened…it did not work. We are now scheduled for a D & C next Tuesday, September 18, 2007 at three o'clock. That's the earliest they could schedule it, since there is no emergency. We did not originally want a D & C, but now, after five days of this, we just need this part to be over and done with. We appreciate everyone who has called/written/e-mailed, and we are asking for more prayer right now until this is done. If all goes well, I'll be home an hour or so after the procedure, and should have an easy (if not speedy) recovery physically.

I was a torrent of emotions by now, but again, all under the surface. Shock at all the options I was given for this. It felt like choosing your own manner of execution. Horrible shame at deciding to have a D & C. Guilt that I had caused us to lose our baby by something I did or did not do. Fear that we'd never conceive again. I felt embarrassment that my predicament was widely known. Worry for my husband who was so focused on me that I worried he would explode in not dealing with his own emotions. Anger that every time I got in the car or turned on the radio that stupid song by Casting Crowns was playing… *every time*! Even body-engulfing agony over losing Peanut and amazing amounts of self-loathing for feeling like I was cheating the world by being "pregnant" but "not pregnant" at the same time.

At its worst, we went to our favorite little Christian coffee shop where we were regulars. They knew we were expecting as well and were always excited for us. This particular day, we went in (in between the medication failure and the scheduled D & C) and ordered breakfast to eat outside and talk. I ordered my food and then my drink, to which the owner gave me a little wink and said, "Decaf of course dear." I was overwhelmed with shame at feeling I was lying by omission in letting him believe I was still pregnant. I was compelled to right this perceived wrong and I blurted out, far too loudly, "No, I don't need decaf anymore!" To his credit, the owner did not bat an eyelash at my outburst and continued taking my husband's order while I tried to invisibly melt my way outside to sit down and hope that no one else heard my horrendous shout of shame.

When my husband came to the table, he said that the owner did in fact catch on to the meaning behind my non-subtle outburst and gave his sincere condolences to us on our loss. I was embarrassed again, and sad that I had ruined this nice man's day. The staff even passed around a card from their bookstore, signed it, and had it ready for us when we checked out. It was very sweet and touching and courteous and I could not get out of there fast enough. I knew I had a neon red sign over my head that said

"Liar, liar pants on fire…I'm not pregnant" and all those little hints for decaf coffee and back pains and needing to pee were big fibs!

The End

The night before the D & C, I picked up yet another prescription I was supposed to take during the night and went to bed, ready for all this to be over with. The next morning I woke up and on the way to the bathroom, realized I was bleeding like a stuck pig. In the few feet from my bed to the bathroom, it soaked through my clothes, was running down both legs, puddling up on the floor, and freaking me and Kevin out quite a lot. I did not have any pain, no cramping, no clots…just bright red blood in large and free flowing quantities. I cleaned myself up, put on a small pillow-version of the maxi-pads and my brave face, and we drove on into Dr. Hayes' office.

When she arrived, I told her of the bleeding and she suggested we do another ultrasound to see where things were. After all, perhaps I finally did miscarry on my own and was done and would not need the D & C. I secretly prayed for that to be true. I also secretly prayed that they would find Peanut still alive, inside me, heart beating fast and strong against all odds and that this would be a miracle of epic proportions. I was terrified of the D & C and not at all looking forward to it so, at the very least, if I could get off the hook with some bleeding and no pain, then all the better.

Unfortunately, the ultrasound confirmed that I had only partially miscarried but it was not complete. That morbidly brought me almost to the point of vomiting right then and there. I had stopped bleeding, but was still dilated and the process unfinished. I was then at risk for an infection which then made the D & C medically necessary. *Of course*, I thought to myself, *I cannot get off this easy now can I. Of course not… and why should I… I should endure each and every humiliation I can pile on.* So on to the D & C process we went.

I will not go into details on that part itself other than to say I hyperventilated halfway through it because I was panicking, and then when it was over and the doctor and nurse left the room, I sat up and finally cried again… sobbed actually. A week had gone by since that fateful day when we learned that Peanut was gone and I had hardly cried beyond that first day. This day though, the dam broke again, and I sobbed uncontrollably and unendingly, seemingly irreparably heartbroken. Even my pouring tears could not have fully emptied my heart from the sadness that had gripped me so tightly. My husband, who had sat there holding my hand through the whole procedure and was my pillar of strength, now sat there holding my head on his chest as I lost the last amount of courage and brave face that I had in me. Peanut was gone––for good now—and I was no longer a mother. No point in hoping for a mistake of some kind or a miracle…what was the point? I was done. This felt finite—like the end of my life at that point—and I did not know how I would survive this. As far as I was concerned, I did not care if I was never going to be a mother again…what was the point when I had failed completely with Peanut. My precious Peanut. My beautiful gray blob. And now, my angel baby.

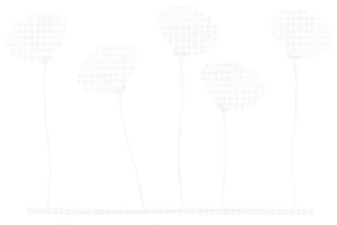

The Aftermath

The days that followed the miscarriage were a blur as well. Another weekend went by with cards, calls, well wishes, and a courtesy meal from that same friend that was brought to us. We skipped church (I could not bear it) and we had planned a follow-up visit with Dr. Hayes in a few weeks to check up on things. Physically, I seemed to heal blessedly quickly. Little bleeding, and as long as I rested and stayed off my feet I had little to no cramping, and it was a reprieve I was glad to have. Emotionally was a different story.

I told myself I needed to jump back into my routines and not wallow too much in my own pity. I went back to work the following Monday. I was a zombie, but was glad to have the diversion and since I worked from home, no one knew I was in sweats and had not showered yet that day. Heck, I might not have bathed for that entire week for all I knew. I was having a lot of trouble sleeping, but insomnia was common for me during my monthly periods and I assumed this was a similar hormonal cause. I called my regular primary care doctor and explained the situation. He expressed his condolences and called me in a one-month prescription of a sleep aid that he said I could take whenever I needed to get me over the rough patch. Once I started that, things seemed to clear up in my head a bit and I started to function on a somewhat more normal, if not numb, level.

One thing I had noticed though, I was tending to easily get headaches for some reason. I would feel fine and then all the sudden, a massive tension headache behind my eyes and sinuses would sink in and about knock me over. I was taking the usual headache medicine, but usually it was not until I got some sleep that night that it would get any better. My mother-in-law was keenly aware of my sleeping concerns and my headaches, and was very worried for me. I could tell because she called and/or e-mailed a lot. Deep down, part of me knew the lack of sleep, the headaches, the fuzzy memory… all of them were symptoms of one main problem: I was not coping with the miscarriage on an emotional level at all. That was one mirror I was not ready to face. I had shut that part of my memory off because I did not want to deal with it… not the pain, the shame, the fear—any of it. I wanted it to go away. In my mind, I had caused Peanut to die and the judgment of my peers was nothing compared to the judgments I had made on myself, and how much more would God have judged me had I taken my cares to Him? I was skipping church, telling myself I was afraid to face all the comments, but that was not true either. I would not talk about it to my husband, and I certainly was not going to talk to *God* about it. Needless to say, God had other plans for my "lack of communication."

When my follow-up visit with Dr. Hayes came, Kevin and I went in and sat down. I was expecting the need to strip down for yet another invasive exam, but she said it was not necessary since I had no further bleeding or cramping. She then asked, simply, "How are *you* doing." I was surprisingly honest, if not vague, in my answer. "Not good," I replied. I told her about the physical stuff, headaches, and difficulty sleeping. At that point, my husband chimed in and ratted me out about the sleeping pills that I had been on for about two-plus weeks solid. She asked what kind and when he told her, she leveled her eyes at me and said in the most serious voice I had ever heard her use, "That stops *right now*." She then turned her level gaze to my husband and said, "Cold

HEATHER D. NELSON

turkey, no discussion." Apparently the prescription I was on was good for the occasional rough night sleep, but not regular use as I had been using it. Kevin had ratted me out on purpose because he was worried about me, and he immediately agreed with the doctor and told her he was glad he said something… the traitor.

She then, returning to her loving/caring self, explained that those pills were not addictive physically, but in the long run would reduce the amount of quality REM sleep I could achieve, and that likely explained a lot of my headaches and stuff. In my mind, I *needed* it to sleep well. She said she knew it would be hard to quit, but it was for the best and I needed to muscle through the rough patch and get past it. For the most part I wanted, in my head, to be healthy. I was okay letting the pills go. They had become a mental crutch more than anything.

I then asked her, as my chin quivered in my effort to hold back tears and my headache came on, "How long am I going to *feel* like this?" Thankfully, she knew I meant emotionally-stunted and was very quick to answer that it could be six weeks or six months, and that there was no time-table or right or wrong answer. I asked her if there was something I could take to help me level out emotionally and she surprisingly said that there was, but she would not prescribe anything for me… yet. Specifically she said, "Miscarriage is a tough thing for anyone to deal with and you need to be kind to yourself and give yourself time to grieve. If in six months you are still feeling as bad as you are now, or if you feel it's beginning to keep you from functioning at work and the rest of your life, then we'll talk about something to help you out. But for now, you are not going through anything abnormal that would raise my concern and I do not think you need any medication."

Outwardly, I was the good patient who agreed with her and we walked out of the office and headed home. Inwardly, I was a little perturbed that I could "expect" to feel *this* crappy for six months and she refused to give me a happy pill to make it all go away. Did she not realize I wanted to get over this *now*? After that appointment, my pleasant *façade* started to crack a bit. And of course, that *song* was playing on the radio nearly every time I got in the car… still! I mean how crazy was the timing that it was the most popular song on the airwaves at that time.

Coping

I went off the sleeping pills as ordered. It was rough for a few nights, but afterward I did start sleeping better on my own. The headaches were still there in my more emotional moments though, but I figured they would work themselves out over time. My husband, who clearly had been talking to his mother, had started asking if I wanted to journal or write to help me "cope" with some of my feelings over the whole thing. I said no. "What for?" I would ask. "There is nothing worth writing over and it would make things worse." He mentioned that it often helped him and others he knew, to get things out in that medium. I blew him off.

Soon thereafter came time for our first trip back to church on Sunday. I was dreading it… completely. I did *not* want to go ever again, but my logic told me it was the best way to try and stay out of hell, so I guess I better go. I knew that the senior pastor had announced our loss to the church for prayer and support, so at least I did not have to tell everyone individually what had happened. But I knew—*knew*—that I would have a dozen or more sad looks on people's faces as they asked that ever popular question, "How ya holdin' up?"

When the day came, I showered, dressed, put on makeup, and primped, and off we went. When we walked in, I immediately sat down for the service and luckily we timed it well and I did not have to chit chat too much. The service was hard. Normally, I was on the worship team singing, but clearly I had taken some time off from that. Singing gave me headaches. But the songs that Sunday were hard and kept bringing tears to my eyes. And I would bet good money that one of the ladies on the team kept looking right at me with sad, puppy dog eyes as she sang one of the songs, as if to say, "This one's for you."

When the music was over, we sat down and made it through the sermon of which I truly do not recall a thing about other than I felt God was talking to me all throughout it. I'm pretty sure the pastor even planned that sermon for that day when he somehow divinely knew I would be there. When the sermon completed, we said our final amens and I proceeded to calmly gather my purse and try to make as speedy an exit as possible. No dice.

HEATHER D. NELSON

My normally very attentive husband had stealthily disappeared that Sunday and was off chatting with some of his buddies. That traitor! Of course, that left me wide open to have not one, not two, but six different women approach me, like a pack of well-coiffed wolves, to tilt their heads, give their best puppy dog eyes, and ask, "How are you feeling?" The cynic in me literally almost laughed at their synchronized sympathy. I told myself inwardly, *They mean well, they are concerned for you, play nice,* and proceeded to give the standard answers. You know the ones, "We're tired, but feeling better, thank you for cards and calls, I'm glad to get this past me, etc." I was hoping my vague, yet polite, answers would be enough to stave off any further digging, and for the most part, it did. I even had one good friend who came to me and said that I looked "very beautiful" that day. It was an unexpected and genuine compliment that I was glad to have. I certainly did not *feel* beautiful, but I could tell she meant it and was grateful that she did not follow that remark up with, "… for someone who killed their baby," which was the atrocious thought in my head. Unfortunately, I had other comments that were less than helpful, to say the least. Below is a very brief listing of some of the more stellar remarks I received then, and over the coming weeks:

- "That is God's way of taking care of the baby because something was wrong with it."
- "I knew someone one time that had like six miscarriages before they had their first baby, it's really common."
- "Sometimes, miscarriage is really for the best."
- "I had a miscarriage once too…" (Then proceed to tell me their personal story, in detail, as if I cared at that moment or had even asked).
- And, my most favorite of all comments that utterly left me speechless: "Did you get to see the pieces of the baby when it came out?"

I knew even then, in my head at least, that these were loving, caring women who were genuinely concerned for me and wanted to comfort me in some way. They wanted to put some rhyme or reason to the loss, or share their stories so I felt less alone, or even tried to reassure me that this was temporary and lots of women go on to have healthy babies after miscarriage. I honestly do not know what the "see the pieces" lady was going for, but I do truly believe even she had a well-meaning, loving intention. But at the time, my heart could not hardly stand it. I was stifled and bitter and had nicely cocooned myself in self-loathing. They asked about the D & C procedure, which I was not prepared to talk about. Their comments made me feel as if they discounted the love I had for Peanut. Like Peanut was not *my* child, but some genetic mistake that God "took care of" for me… aren't I lucky. I felt invaded and naked and totally stripped of my defenses by some remarks that I was not prepared for.

Sadly, this carried out of the church and into the rest of my life. Family and friends would say things, meaning well, that my heart would twist and turn into some horrible shard of glass to dig yet another scar. And every time, my head would throb as I tried to stifle my looks of shock and cynical comments, and keep the calm outer face on and… get through it.

I began to dread church a little and withdraw from everything. I did not have the emotional energy to protect myself anymore, and it felt that I would snap at anyone for anything. I did not want to be hateful to others, so retreat seemed the easiest route. Of course that is not true either… I did not care about others as much as I cared about me… I was hurting, and withdrawal seemed easier than dealing.

I should note that during this difficult time, it was not all bad… there were some bright spots in there that I held on to for dear life and still remember. For example, one friend of ours who had suffered two miscarriages in her life brought us dinner twice the week of the actual D & C. In one of those, she included a card that simply said, "This is crappy and awful and sucks, and I'm sorry you have to go through this. We'll pray for you both." I literally laughed at that because it was *exactly* how I felt! It was crappy and it *was* awful and it *did* suck! I loved her a little bit more for her candid card and caring gesture, and for her inability to serve up platitudes that meant nothing.

Another elderly widower in our church bumped into us at our coffee shop. While Kevin was grabbing our drinks, this nice man sat at my table, firmly grabbed my hand, and said, "I was real sorry to hear about your loss... my wife and I lost a baby one time and I remember it was real hard on her. I'll pray for you guys." Then he got up and left. It was bliss. No forced platitudes to make me or him feel better, no detailed story about how his wife lost her baby, not even a token, "God planned this" remark. Just genuine concern, an offer for prayer, and then he left us alone. It was heavenly. I was not forced to talk about it or comfort *him* in any way... I only had to silently accept his kindness. Of course, on the heels of feeling such sympathy for something that clearly had affected him for decades, I panicked a little. Would I one day be the little old lady still mourning my miscarried baby? Would my life forever be shaped by this malignant event, and would I ever be able to let this go? I envisioned myself as a little old lady, hearing of some young couples loss, and selfishly grieving myself for my own loss. I was proactively castigating myself for selfishness I had intended in the coming ages of my life!

Family was another area that had its good and bad moments. One of my sister-in-laws had suffered a miscarriage prior to her first baby as well, and she expressed her sadness and then, in a later chat, mentioned that she hoped we did not "un-enjoy" our next pregnancy out of fear. I appreciated her input and her positive thinking that we would actually have another shot at this, but did not put too much stock in it at the time. My stepmother was never able to have children of her own and when she and I talked, she was genuinely grieving with me. It was nice to have someone who did not "blow off" my pain, but sometimes it was overwhelming too because I felt compelled to comfort her at times. Nothing she said or did, mind you, just me feeling that way. Sometimes her tears with me were welcome, and others they were a reminder that I had failed this pregnancy for the both of us.

Other family would make the typical comments that meant well, but hurt deeply. Even my mother who loves me forever had some hurtful times unintentionally. One bright spot was my dear cousin, who had never been pregnant at the time. She asked honest questions and gave me a wonderful chance to talk *not* about the death, but the life—the pregnancy itself. Not overly invasive questions about the D & C, but rather asked about the pregnancy and how it felt. It was nice to have someone acknowledge in that way that Peanut was more than a medical procedure. It felt like I was getting to talk about the good stuff before the loss for a change, and I needed that.

Those good moments I had, I held on to, and the hurtful ones I tried to let go of while mentally making a note of who I could and could not talk to based on my moods. Little did I know the real work that God intended for me had not begun yet.

Closure

By now, nearly a month or more had gone by since the D & C procedure. I had attended church about two times maybe, and had declined to be in the worship team because I could not handle singing without getting headaches. I was withdrawing from nearly everything and still suffering from an erratic sleep schedule. The headaches were growing worse. I can remember vividly asking my small group to pray for my lack of sleep and the headaches. Even after all that "healing time" I had given myself, I was still not feeling any better, and my mother-in-law––love her—was still calling, e-mailing, and checking in on me. And sure enough, that song—that stupid song—was still playing on the radio every time I got in the car. Like some morbid top ten hit reminding me of my dead baby and my failure at the most basic God-given ability I had as a woman.

One day, two friends and I were chatting and the topic of miscarriage came up. One of my friends was in school to be a counselor and had a miscarriage of her own. I was grateful to listen to her input. I was honest that I was not coping at all, but really did not know how. My counselor friend mentioned that I had to "feel the grief" and get through it. My other friend, who I consider a spiritual giant, talked about taking it to God and letting His Word lead me through the rough times. She even specifically mentioned reading and praying through the book of Psalms to help see the character of God. Both of those clicked for me as two things I had not done. No wait, that's not right. Both of those things clicked for me as two things I did not know *how* to do.

I realized at that moment that I had never lost anyone close to me. Both my parents were living, and the only grandparents who had died at that time either were largely unknown to me or died very early in my life and I had no chance to know them. I did not know how to grieve, much less grieve with God leading me through it. Truth be told, I did not much want God to be a part of my grieving. I did not deserve it. I wish, after the fact, I had felt differently and listened, but I did not. At the time, I felt a little angry at the whole situation, as well as confused and lost, and all I wanted was to "be okay" on my own and not take my shame or pain to Him. I had not once stopped to consider *how* to be okay.

About this time, my mother-in-law made one of her infamous calls that are perfectly timed when you do not want to share, but need to, and God clearly knows better than you, so there! We chatted and she too confirmed that you have to just go through the grief; you have to feel it. I admitted to her that I did not know how because I had never done it. She then said, "It's different for different people. Some people write to express themselves, and for others, it's music. You have to find something—for you—to help you bring those feelings to the surface, so you can feel them and get them out. That will probably get rid of your headaches too and help you sleep, to unclog all those emotions you have been stuffing." I knew by that last part that my darling traitor husband had been ratting me out again, but I also knew she was right. I finally admitted to myself that it was time.

"Praise You In This Storm"

I was sure by now
God You would have reached down
And wiped our tears away
Stepped in and saved the day
But once again, I say "Amen," and it's still raining

As the thunder rolls
I barely hear Your whisper through the rain
"I'm with you"
And as Your mercy falls
I raise my hands and praise the God who gives
And takes away

And I'll praise You in this storm
And I will lift my hands
For You are who You are
No matter where I am
And every tear I've cried
You hold in Your hand
You never left my side
And though my heart is torn
I will praise You in this storm

I remember when
I stumbled in the wind
You heard my cry to you
And you raised me up again
My strength is almost gone
How can I carry on
If I can't find You

But as the thunder rolls
I barely hear You whisper through the rain
"I'm with you"
And as Your mercy falls
I raise my hands and praise the God who gives
And takes away

HEATHER D. NELSON

I lift my eyes unto the hills
Where does my help come from?
My help comes from the Lord
The Maker of heaven and earth
And I'll praise You in this storm
And I will lift my hands
For You are who You are
No matter where I am
And every tear I've cried
You hold in Your hand
You never left my side
And though my heart is torn
I will praise You in this storm
And though my heart is torn
I will praise You in this storm

The following Monday, in early October, was our small group night and I attended alone since Kevin had to work late. We had two new people attending our group, which perturbed me a bit personally for no good reason. They were the associate pastor candidate and his wife, visiting and seeing if they liked the church, etc. I was irritated because I did not feel comfortable discussing my need for miscarriage prayer in front of strangers. I was polite and quiet, and when prayer request time came I vaguely mentioned that I had not felt well and was still struggling with sleeping and headaches, and could use some prayer. The pastoral candidate and his wife blissfully did not ask any questions, and the rest of the group knowingly nodded their heads that they understood. I loved my small group for that.

Later, as I was driving in the dark, I turned on the radio. Lo and behold, that song—*that annoyingly persistent song*—was playing on the radio. Then I realized it was not on the radio. My darling husband, in all his infinite God-given wisdom, had burned the song onto a CD for me. That loving, wonderful, traitorous man of mine whom I love dearly. I decided to give in a bit and listen to the song. I tried…I really did.

But I could not listen without crying, which then gave me a headache, so I shut it off.

Then, while driving in the dark on the quiet street, I spoke to God. Not prayer really, rather I just started talking to God and telling Him that I did not understand what He wanted. I was angry, hurt, and scared, and I felt like He was leaving me floundering out here with no support. I expressed my frustration that if He had planned to be subtle and help me covertly, I was not catching on and He needed to be a bit more obvious. I even asked for Him to send some burning bush of a sign to me so I would know what He wanted me to do.

Alas, no shrubbery caught fire and I pulled into my garage and shut the car off, still as lost as ever. Instead of sucking up my feelings and going in the house, I sat there. I could not go in upset like I was but did not know what to do and for once I could not stop the tears. I could not block up the dam; it had cracked and would not be repaired it seemed.

Finally, with no small amount of prompting from the Spirit, I put that CD in and turned on the song and sat there in the dark listening to it on repeat mode. Over and over. And I began to sing it. Or rather, I began to cry/sing simultaneously and sound like a drowning wildebeest. The lyrics were cutting. "*I was sure by now… You would have reached down and wiped my tears away,*" "*My strength is almost gone, how can I carry on if I can't find You.*" It was as if those lyrics were written for me, for Peanut, for this loss and this time in my life. A song that previously my husband and I had attributed to our great triumph over perceived infertility had become the swan song of my grief and pain and most dark time. As I listened to it over and over in my garage—in the car, in the dark—I cried and sang and somewhere in that time, my heart turned. What started out as tears and hurt and pain became prayers and grief. I began begging God to help me. I cried and cried and poured every horrible thought and emotion I had been stuffing at the feet of my Lord. My headache was nowhere to be found and the tears were freely flowing down my face. I had somehow unblocked the emotion and finally given up to God all my grief and hurt and confusion and anger and pain and simply pleaded for Him to "step in and save the day." I admitted fully that I did not understand why this had happened, but that I needed Him to pull me through it because I could not do it on my own. I could not cope, could not heal, and could not "get over it" without God's personal involvement, and I was pleading with Him to carry me through. I admitted that I *wanted* to be okay again, but I could not find my way out of the maze. I asked God not to leave me alone…little did I know He was always there for me and was waiting for me to realize it.

After that, I went into the house and instead of going to see my husband or plop down in front of the TV, I sat down at my computer and typed a long awaited letter to Peanut.

Dear Peanut

Part of me inside was slightly kicking myself for taking so long to finally take the advice that was given to me a month prior. It was the final turning point for me. I realized through all my hurt and confusion and issues with God, I was grief-stricken *on behalf of* Peanut. As Peanut's mother, I was terrified that he had suffered somehow, or that he had physically hurt in his process of dying. I feared that after his death, all that time still in my body had somehow blocked him from moving on to heaven. I was sorry that all that had happened to him. What's worse, I was afraid that he did not know how much we loved and wanted him, and I was scared beyond words that we would somehow forget him and he would be looking down on us from heaven knowing that he "did not count" somehow. I realized then, that I wanted him to know how very much we adored that precious baby, no matter how small he was or how short his time was with us. I wanted him to know how honored I was to be able to carry him inside of me, even if for a few short weeks. I wanted him to know that he would never *ever* leave my heart, and that no matter the lack of title to the real world, I would always feel like a mommy because of the gift he gave me: to have shared what tiny life he had with me. All of this and more I poured into the following letter to our baby.

Dear Peanut,

I'm not really sure why I'm writing this letter to you. I know that you do not need it, you cannot read it where you are anyway, and you would not need to read it, as you have a far greater understanding of what has happened than I. I know you are in heaven, with God. I know you are in a far more beautiful and perfect place, and that you are waiting for the day to come when we get to meet you face-to-face. I know you love us, and I know you feel our love too. But all these things I know…in my head…have not managed to yet heal the hurt in my heart.

Your daddy and I prayed hard for you. We prayed to God regularly to bring us a baby…to heal mommy and daddy's infertility, and to bless us with a child we could love. We visited all the doctors and specialists that we could, trying to "help God" to help mommy get pregnant. The doctors did not give us very good odds, but we kept praying. And then, it happened. A positive test result! We were excited, even daddy, that we called all our family that night to tell them of your impending arrival.

We spent the next twelve weeks in utter bliss. We loved knowing you were on your way, and we planned so many things. Mommy was planning the nursery, decorating, clothing, and scrapbooks. Daddy was planning for financial changes, vacation before your arrival, and the daddy-baby dates the two of you would have. We did not know if you were a boy or a girl…so we called you Peanut. That was about the shape you were on our sonogram picture, so it just stuck. I hope you liked it. The whole family, before long, called you Peanut too. Papaw in Mississippi, Papa in Washington, even your Nana, Noni, and aunt and uncles all called you Peanut. They would call us and ask, "How's Peanut?" We could not wait to see you and know you more. Mommy thanked God every night for the wonderful blessing of you. It did not matter that she was a little more tired, or a little more sore, or a little more hungry than usual. She was so excited to know you were coming and just could not wait to see the real evidence of you—her growing belly and feeling you kick.

But these dreams were not meant to be. At our twelve week checkup, the doctor could not find your heartbeat. She used a Doppler, a sonogram, and an ultrasound—everything she could. Finally, when she did find you, she told us that she was really sorry, but that we'd lost you. I could see your tiny body on the monitor…you were still there, still my Peanut…but your little heart had stopped beating and you had not grown in weeks. Mommy was in shock and could not believe it. Your daddy was there too. He came to every appointment for you and was strong for mommy while we were in the office…but even he broke down once we got to the car. We could not believe you were gone and we did not know how we would go on. You were not just "a baby." You were our baby. You were not the "it" inside of me. You were Peanut, our child, who we had begged God to send us.

Over the next week, even though your little body had died, Mommy's body would not let go. I wanted desperately to keep you inside, safe, and I could not seem to complete the process that was intended. We were really heartbroken at the prospect of losing you, but also anxiously awaiting the final moment when you would leave Mommy's body. It was so hard. So we decided to let the doctor's help us. We did medication, and finally a D & C. Please know, that we never wanted to lose you. Ever. We were not wanting to remove you quickly because we did not love you, and if there was any way at all that we could have saved you, we would have. I worried that you suffered during that time. I worried that you were in pain or hurting somehow. We just needed to move beyond that one step, toward some kind of closure, but I promise, we did not want to lose you.

I still am so sad over losing you. I cry every day when thinking of all the things I cannot have with you. I'll never see my belly growing and know Peanut is inside of me. I'll never feel you kick and move. I'll never complain of the indigestion you may have caused me, or the way my clothes will not fit. Your daddy will never talk to you through my belly, never sing you songs like he planned. All our friends will never throw a shower to honor you. Our families will never make the drive to meet you when you finally arrive. Mommy and Daddy will never get to see your little face when you are born, hold you in our arms, see what all our love and prayers have made. We'll never hear you laugh, or cry, or giggle. We'll never see your expressions as you learn about new foods. I'll never feel that close bond with you when breastfeeding in the night. Daddy will never get to nap with you on his chest. No one will ever get to see your baby book and how you've grown. You'll never play with all your cousins. We're sad at all the beautiful things we'll miss because you did not make it. Things like your first Christmas, when you would be old enough to eat all the wrapping paper and play with the bows, but utterly ignore the gifts inside. Things like your first bath, as you squiggled and wormed around all slippery, and mommy and daddy tried to hold on to you and get you clean. Seeing you play with Bailey, our dog. Your first little curl of your hair, your first tooth. All the things we would cherish and all the memories we would save for your whole life. Those are gone now.

If I could talk to you right now, I would have many things to say. Are you okay? Did you hurt at all when you inside me? Was there anything I could have done to ease your pain and comfort you? Did you know how very much we loved you? Do you know still how much we love you? Do you understand that even though we are trying to move on, it's not because we want to forget you? We love you so very much, and we cannot imagine why you cannot be with us. We know that God has a reason, but it's hard to see and understand that right now. I'm sad not to have you with me. I hate that I cannot feel you inside me and I wish so badly that I could just know you were okay, know you did not hurt. I felt guilty for having you "stuck" inside me, but now I feel guiltier for having asked the doctor to help get you out. I hope you know that all my decisions during that time were not ever an attempt to "get rid of you." That was never what we wanted. In fact, right up until the D & C, I wondered, "What if?" What if Peanut's not dead? What if there is something else we can do? But I guess you were really in God's hands and not ours. And He was always in control. That's been hard for mommy… not having the control to understand why you could not stay with us.

If I could talk to God face-to-face right now, I would ask for a glimpse of what would have been. What would mommy and daddy be like when you were born? What kind of baby would you have been? What kind of personality would you have as you grew up? Would you be musical like mommy, or more logical and technical like daddy? Would you make friends easily and be social, or be more of a loner who preferred quiet things? Would you be a good driver, and which of us would be brave enough to teach you? Who would your first kiss be with? Would you go to college? Who would you choose to marry and start your own life with? Of course, no matter what God showed me during this glimpse, I would be proud to see who you would have become. No matter what you turned out like, we would love you just as much as we love you now, if not more. If I could talk to God, I would ask to understand why, but then again, who would not? I would ask if you were okay right now, and if you knew how much we wanted you? And I would ask that God please hug you, every day, and tell you He loved you, just like we would if you were here. And we would, you know… we would have hugged and kissed you every day and told you we loved you, so you would never ever have doubted how important and special you were to us.

I miss you so much every day. I'm sad that you are not here. I'm sad that you were just not strong enough to make it all the way. But even with all the sadness in my heart right now, I'm still so grateful. I'm glad I had you at all—I'm glad I got to see your little body and your little heartbeat on the first sonogram. I'm glad that Daddy and everyone loved you and knew you as Peanut… and not "it."

I want you to know one more thing, and it's important. Mommy and Daddy are going to keep trying again to have another baby. We plan to start as soon as we can, and we'll try and pray as hard as we did for you. But that does not mean for one second that we love you any less, or that our hearts did not break to lose you. We want a family, that has not changed, but I would give anything right now to have that family start with you. God has other plans, which you may now understand better than us since you are with Him. I feel compelled to reassure you that our efforts to heal and move on and try again and on are not at all a reflection of our feelings for you.

I think I may always have a special place in my heart just for you. And what's more, I think we'll remember you as our first/oldest baby. You will always hold a place of honor for us, and that is not at all diminished by any of this that has happened. We love you with all our hearts and we hope, more than anything, that you know that right now. If you have a moment to ask God for us, please ask for a hug, and please ask for a little grace for us too. Mommy's not doing very well right now, and she could use some heavenly help. Say hello to your great-great granddads, both of them. I'm sure they'll keep you in good company until we see you.

> All our love forever,
> Mommy and Daddy.

While I typed (then, and now for that matter), I cried. I cried and cried and cried and cried. It was, to date, the most heartfelt piece of work I had ever created in my lifetime. When it was over, and I was done, I cleaned myself up a bit, printed it, and gave it to my husband to read. He read it and cried, and said it was everything he would have said himself. I felt some peace knowing that I was not alone in my crazy paranoid fears and I wished I would have shared it with him sooner. I then found an empty box and proceeded to put all the cards, gifts, baby books, sonogram pictures, positive pregnancy tests, and that letter inside. I then shoved the box to the top of the guest room closet, closed the door, and went to bed to sleep the best I had slept ever since that fateful day this all began.

I did not have this scripture at the time to draw from, but wished I had. "You saw me before I was born. Every day of my life was recorded in Your book. Every moment was laid out before a single day had passed. How precious are your thoughts about me, Oh God" (Psalm 139:16–17, NLT). Perhaps it would have allayed my fears to know that God was closely watching over Peanut through all of this, but at the time I was clueless.

Finding Peace

After that night, I seemed to recover a little bit in a different way. I rejoined the worship team and took up my decorating committee responsibilities as well. I began picking up my regular steam at work again and started to feel a bit more like myself. I still had my emotional moments and a few rough patches, but was feeling more and more like I had turned a corner and was ready to try again for another baby. Sure enough, my body thought the same thing and my cycles began normally. We jumped back in, both feet first, into trying to conceive. We also planned a little vacation, just the two of us. We technically had not had a true vacation since our honeymoon and had wanted to do this anyway, but now it was more of a "get to know each other again" trip to rekindle our couple-hood after all the emotion and mess of the miscarriage. Timing wise, it was fairly perfect since my intense 150mg per day doses of Clomid ended and ovulation occurred on the trip. We had lots of time for "vacation festivities" as it were, and I was really ready for a getaway to hopefully feel human again.

The vacation was great. We did a little over a week tour driving from Idaho to Seattle, WA, with a pit stop in Dayton, WA along the way. In Seattle, we did ferry rides, shopping, the Wharf, caught a show at the Fifth Avenue Playhouse, and even did dinner at the Space Needle. Kevin was back on his home soil, which he loved, and I was getting a nice "escape" from life which I needed. We laughed, and loved, and we had fun. In all ways possible, it was a perfect vacation. I remembered, too, how much I loved my husband. Of course, the reprieve was a small one because then the real work began, but it was perfect nonetheless, and I was relaxed for the first time in a long time.

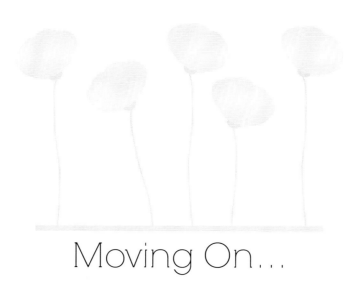

Moving On...

The months of November and December 2007, as well as January and February 2008, were all failed attempts to recapture the lightning in a jar we had with Peanut. Kevin wanted to try things semi-naturally, as we had before, thinking we could get lucky again. In fact, he was downright convinced that if we did it once, we could do it again. And, in his mind, why spend all that money for IUI if we did *not* need to? My husband... ever the frugal pragmatist. We also lightly revisited the adoption discussion. I was panicking a little and thinking we could do *both* adoption *and* try to conceive on our own, but Kevin was not ready for adoption. We set that aside, again, and moved forward with our own efforts. Dr. Hayes increased my Clomid to 100mg per day each cycle. I ovulated, we "did the deed" as per the instructions, and still could not get pregnant. Even with all that extra medicinal help that we did not need before, I could not get pregnant.

Month after month went by with no luck. My spirits were crushed (or I thought at the time) and I was utterly discouraged. In my mind, we had long passed that time of "lots of people get pregnant quickly after a miscarriage," as well as zoomed right past that "we did it before, we can do it again" mentality. I was withdrawing more and more from my social calendar and beginning to struggle again. Most of my battle was internal at this point and I was fully blaming myself for all our problems.

My darling husband, who grew up with two loving parents that stayed married to each other and raised their children with good Christian values in good Christian schools, never did a thing wrong in his life. As such, he was a perfect golden example of someone who should be "loved by God" in my eyes. I, on the other hand, was a picture of near catastrophe for most of my childhood. My parents were divorced, and I was intelligent and well-mannered on the surface, but an utter wild child underneath and would push the envelope about as far as it would go every chance I got. I was convinced that all our fertility problems, the miscarriage, all of it… were my fault. And why should they not be? After all, my near perfect husband who had read and studied more of the Bible than I ever dreamed, and who considered his church youth pastor to be his best friend in high school, could not possibly be the reason that God is sitting up on His cloud smiting our family planning efforts. Oh no, that would be *all* my fault for the bad friends, worse choices, wild parties, and embarrassing run-ins with police that should have (but miraculously never did) end me up on that show, *Cops*! At least, that was my thinking at the time. I was harshly judging myself and praying fervently each day for God to forgive my multitude of sins. I would plead with God to not use my transgressions to punish my husband who was undeserving of such castigation. I also began a carefully worded begging series of prayers along the lines of "Please, please, please, please." You never know how *one more please* might do the trick after all. I begged God like this for quite awhile, in fact. Apparently God was listening to my wildly repetitive prayers and decided to finally answer them… at least in part.

Forgiven and Loved

Now, before you jump to the conclusion that God blessed us with another pregnancy at that point, let me squash that hope right now. That was not the part of the prayer God chose to answer. However, He did decide to address my guilt and self-flagellation about all this infertility stuff.

It took a few months, but the first huge leap was our pastor's well-timed sermon series on grace and justification. As it happens, I had always struggled with forgiveness. Both forgiving others that had hurt me, as well as accepting forgiveness for myself when I had wronged another. In fact, if I realized I had hurt someone I loved, I would bend over backward trying to *make* it better. Any little acts of retribution that I felt were necessary to right the wrong and assuage my own guilt was paramount for any indiscretion I felt I had committed. Often times, I would go far over and beyond what some would call necessary to make myself feel better. And sometimes even for wrongs I did *not* think I had done, but had been accused for, and other times, wrongs I *saw* that I had done, but no one else believed or accounted me for. In general, when I screwed up, I felt the need to *work* it off. Likewise, if someone wronged me, I felt they had to *work* to earn back my trust or affection or whatever had been lost. I would even often times get bitter if I felt someone had *not* worked hard enough or for long enough to feel their contrition. That was the crux of the issue for me. I wanted others to *feel* how sorry I was, and I wanted to *feel* how sorry they were in return.

> 22 This righteousness from God comes through faith in Jesus Christ to all who believe. There is no difference, 23 for all have sinned and fall short of the glory of God, 24 and are justified freely by his grace through the redemption that came by Christ Jesus. 25 God presented him as a sacrifice of atonement, through faith in his blood. He did this to demonstrate his justice, because in his forbearance he had left the sins committed beforehand unpunished- 26 he did it to demonstrate his justice at the present time, so as to be just and the one who justifies those who have faith in Jesus.
>
> 27 Where, then, is boasting? It is excluded. On what principle? On that of observing the law? No, but on that of faith. 28 For we maintain that a man is justified by faith apart from observing the law.
>
> Romans 3:21–28 (NIV).

I had taken that same narrow-minded concept and put it to play here. Here where I felt an entire lifetime of fun-loving sinning I had done in my younger and more oat-sowing days. I was certain those wild oats had irreparably damaged my chances at being a mother. I did not think I could ever work to earn back God's good graces... or my husband's, for that matter. I guess, looking back, considering that I did *not* die from any of my sins, I figured being struck with infertility was *my* punishment. However, I was not alone in this game. My, seemingly, perfect sinless husband was in this mess with me. Thus, in my twisted, overworked logic, *I had caused not only my own suffering and pain, but had now caused the pain and anguish of the man I loved most on this earth!*

It was amazing how far my twisted, worrywart thinking got me. No wonder I was withdrawing from my social circle and becoming more depressed. Each month that went by without a positive pregnancy test was another confirmation, in my mind, of exactly how bad I was in the eyes of God. It was also putting a bit of a wedge between my husband and I. Not a huge wedge, but a silent sliver of space between us. My remorse at dragging him down with me was suffocating. I did not feel right sharing with him my struggles or feelings on all this baby-making mess. Likewise, I kept waiting for him to throw his hands up and say, "You know what, I said I would always love you and cherish you and honor you, but that has never been tested until now and you are suddenly very hard to love, so I'm outta here."

This guilt was growing into a massive and burdensome cloud over my life. And with all the additional stressors I had piled on myself, this guilt was one problem God had in his sights to deal with. And it all started with that well-timed sermon series on grace and justification. It was a multi-week series by which our pastor described the entire biblical basis for why God's grace covered all our sins, in full, by the single act of His son's death on the cross. As such, by believing and accepting in that death, we were totally forgiven. I listened each week and took notes and was enjoying the series but truthfully still could not get it. I could not understand how God could totally love and forgive me considering how bad I was. I knew that if God actually knew how awful I was, He'd scratch my name of his big book right then and there. For that matter, I also *knew* that if my friends and family knew how awful I truly was, they'd disown me in full.

Then, one Sunday, the pastor was wrapping up his sermon and referenced a portion of scripture that hit me like a ton of bricks. The whole series centered around the book of Romans, but in particular, this jumped out at me. "This righteousness from God comes through faith in Jesus Christ to *all* who believe. There is no difference, for *all* have sinned and fallen short of the glory of God, and *all* are justified freely by his grace through the redemption that came by Jesus Christ." I read that and it finally clicked in my tiny pea brain. *All* are forgiven. Not all who have to work really hard for it, or all have to *earn* their good graces back before stepping foot beyond the pearly gates. No. All are forgiven, by accepting Jesus' sacrifice for us. And not forgiven for the little stuff, but *all* are forgiven *no matter the sin*! It said it right there in black and white, "There is no difference for all have sinned." It did not matter how big the sin was in my mind or in reality, it was forgiven. In short, this righteousness is from God, and there is *no* matter or difference what sin was committed, for *all* are freely justified by His grace. And then the light bulb finally came on and, in my mind, the subtext was, *Duh, Heather, it's sitting here waiting on you this whole time; you only need to accept it.*

It was an amazing epiphany for me to finally realize this small being verb: "*are* forgiven." Wow, that meant that my infertility was not some arbitrary punishment doled out by a vengeful God for my past sins, and that also meant that my infertility was not punishing my husband either. Hmm… interesting concept to wrap my brain around. I clearly had to rethink some of my own theories on why all this was happening to us. I was so excited to finally understand God's forgiveness and acceptance of me overall, that I failed to realize how significantly it applied to my then current struggles.

"Oh, but wait," I could hear God saying, "There's more!" If I could so easily accept God's forgiveness for the seemingly awful things I had done, then how much more so did I owe my forgiveness and compassion to others? And not that surface level kind of forgiveness where you *say* you forgive someone and hold on to your anger… but *really* forgive them deep down in your core. The potential for my relationships with friends and family instantly took on a huge new dimension. I could not imagine how much my guard would now be lowered since I would no longer be hanging on to perceived slights. I knew that this would not be an instant fix for my soul, but this understanding was a huge leap in the right direction, and I was spiritually psyched to see how it would move my life.

Finally Communicating

Now, about this time, my mother-in-law had another fortuitously timed, but irritatingly accurate, phone heart-to-heart with me. She called and checked in on me periodically to see how I was doing, and mostly I would give her the standard vague answers and statistical data I gave everyone else. But this one particular phone call stuck out to me as being God-sent as well. We actually got into the discussion of how I felt like I could not openly talk to my husband about all this stuff, because I kept waiting on the other shoe to drop with him. And I confessed to her that I was sure he would walk out on me or say "no more" to our family efforts. My mother-in-law, always gentle when being deadly accurate, stated that she completely understood my fears. After all, my own mother had been divorced multiple times during my childhood, and each divorce or remarriage would come with a residential move and sometimes school change. I had no long history of stability there. I myself had one failed marriage under my belt before meeting my now wonderful husband, and there was no shortage of friendships that had left me high and dry as well. It was totally understandable, she said, for me to have those fears. Then—ever so gently—she said me, "But you have to stop putting that fear on Kevin and let that go, right now." Just that blunt. She proceeded to tell me that enough time had passed (years) for me to experience Kevin's character both as a man and a husband. She said it was high time for me to stop comparing him to all my past failed relationships. She went on to instruct me that when those negative thoughts crept in, I needed to push them aside and remember that Kevin did not deserve to be judged as a side-by-side comparison to past failures of people no longer in my life. Talk about a loving and gentle call to the carpet, or, as we call them in my house, a come to Jesus meeting!

I immediately felt more than a little guilty for having done exactly what she said I was doing. I was expecting my husband to fail me, as past people had, and in so doing was not only disrespecting his character and integrity, but also putting him into a no-win situation. Since I would never fully trust him as my partner in life, how could I ever fully let him *lead* me or our family, as the Bible calls husbands to lead. I was tying my husband's hands by withholding the respect and full-on trust that he deserved from me. As all this was rattling around in my head, I immediately recalled the sermon message that *all* sins *are* forgiven, and that I did not deserve to be failed in that way, nor did my husband deserve to be judged by other's mistakes or sins. My head was starting to hurt from all this "clicking" going on, but it finally jarred an important conversation between Kevin and I.

I finally, tearfully, admitted that I felt like he was not 100 percent with me in our family planning efforts. I felt that he was tagging along for the ride—and that any minute now, I was afraid he would jump ship on me for being too hard to love.

Likewise, I admitted that I felt more alone because I did not think I could share things with him for this same aforementioned fear. I am sure, through all the tears and snot and sobbing, that I said a lot of other confessional-like things, but the end result was a mix of apology to him and asking for acceptance from him at the same time. My darling husband immediately alleviated all my fears and reaffirmed all my faith in him by saying all the right things at all the right times. Truth be told, I do not recall verbatim what he said, but the important thing was that I was finally letting go of some of this self-inflicted guilt over our family struggles, and was removing that wedge to bring us back to a place that I felt more like partners in this struggle. We also discussed the adoption issue and his lack of enthusiasm to even look into it. He admitted that he really wanted a genetic connection to our child. He wanted and dreamed of the comments like, "Your baby has your wife's eyes," and "Wow, your son looks like you." He was not prepared emotionally to let those dreams go and was afraid he would not bond as well with an adopted child. It was a brutally honest answer that he gave me, and I loved him for sharing it with me. I felt a huge honor to be trusted with such a large truth of his. This little "chat" of ours was the motherload of turning points in our marriage. We were instantly closer, and I felt that we had bonded on a level that had not existed prior to all this. I also gained a newfound respect for him as a husband. I loved his vulnerability and honesty, and it made me trust him more with my own feelings. I began to feel more confident that I was not alone in my want for a family. I also realized that we truly *were* a family of two and that we just might survive this no matter what the outcome was. And as if all this was not enough, God decided this was a good time to tackle another stress demon that had plagued our marriage from the very beginning: money.

The Almighty Dollar

Shortly after this spiritual epiphany downpour, our church began a new money series called Financial Peace University. It was created and hosted by Dave Ramsey and lasted about thirteen weeks. We both felt strongly that we needed to take part in this. Though the ninety-eight dollar class fee was a little much for us, we found a way to make it happen so we could go. In fact, our entire small group decided to take this class together, which turned out to be a huge support system for what would prove to be some big lifestyle changes.

The class was extremely educational on the basics of money management, but moreover gave us invaluable tools to come together as a couple and discuss our financial goals, and our financial future. We had an ongoing debt cycle that we desperately needed to get under control. Shamefully, I will admit we were well over twenty thousand dollars in the hole from various debtors, credit cards, and such. Beyond the debt, we were never a unified couple in our approach to spending. My husband was the tight-fisted saving nazi, and I was the free-spirited work hard/play hard/spend hard wife. While we wanted the same end goal, we were often two warring parties pulling opposite ends of the same rope. Add to that tension the stress of medical costs and infertility, and the huge pit in the middle was deep and wide and *growing*.

Using Dave Ramsey's tools and our small group's support, we were able to put into action some quick steps that alleviated our financial struggle significantly. We saved up a small sum of cash, we paid off major debt, and generally we learned how to live on a smaller budget without feeling restricted. We left money stress in the past and began to reshape the way we handled our finances as a couple, with responsible planning and fewer emotional weak moments of frenzied spending. Or as Dave Ramsey says, we had taken a step towards "Living like no one else." Debt was the surprising norm in our society, but it did not have to be the ruling party in our home, as we learned. We made a choice, that even with our family planning hopes and dreams, we would not let all these emotions force us into bad financial decisions that would haunt us for years. Yes, infertility was expensive and could potentially be an unsuccessful cost to bear, but at least we had been handed the tools to now handle those expenses wisely. Moreover, our small group was riding the "debt free train" with us. That meant we had even more support to help strengthen not only our spiritual walk with the Lord, but our marital walk without debt. All in all, the class was phenomenal and I wish I could have packaged Dave Ramsey up and sent him to all my family and friends!

This class was one more way that we were growing as a couple and coming together to partner up against the tough stuff. I really felt our relationship was growing stronger. Many of my fears and my husband's frustrations were easing up quite a bit as we continued our family planning efforts. Even with all these huge relationship "wins," however, the end of 2007 and beginning of 2008 were medically marked by multiple failed attempts to conceive. Over and over we tried… and over and over we failed. Our hearts were still heavy with sorrow over our childless state. Dr. Hayes increased my Clomid to 100mg per day each cycle, and the side effects increased with it. I ovulated each time and we did a little "baby dancing" as per the instructions and still could not manage to conceive. Each month, despite our new unified front in our marriage, my heart would break a little more that I was not, again, a mother. Those fears of never again feeling that joy of a positive pregnancy test got bigger and bigger. The primary difference this time around, however, was that after months of repeated failure, I did not shove my fears down and keep silent… I spoke with my husband. I was somewhat relieved when even he admitted that he felt it was time to try a little more intervention. He and I agreed that IUI was in order. It was the first time, since we began our family journey, that we had the same feelings at the same time and wanted the same path. With that irony in full bloom, back to Dr. Greer's we went.

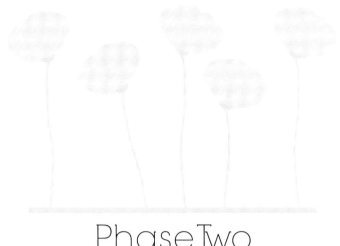

Phase Two

Clomid had been about as much fun as a root canal, sans Novocain, but it was relatively low, on the medical world scale, of options to try. We knew we had just begun dipping our toes into the treatments available to us. We had not tried much more than good old-fashioned "timed intercourse" either, for that matter, and as of February, we had officially been trying for over a year. In fact, we had been trying officially for fifteen months and during that time we had found very little success and one major heart-wrenching failure. I had to catch my breath when I realized that sad statistic. After *fifteen months* of trying, we had not even begun to take advantage of all the options medical science had for us to pursue. Sure, prior to this we had been trying to conceive, but until now we were not technically classified as "infertile." We now had that proud badge of honor to wear. That was some seriously heavy reality. After twelve consecutive months of failed attempts at conception, we could now walk into any doctor's office and clinically be called "infertile." To quote the late great Chris Farley, "Well, *lah- dee- freaking- dah!*"

Armed with this depressing information, both Kevin and I agreed that it was time for more help and perhaps some more major medical intervention. The fact that we were both on the same page was a change for us. Since we had embarked on this journey, our relationship had begun to mature in a lot of ways. Having our marriage tested in such a way had done a lot for our communication, and even more for my trust in Kevin… and in God too for that matter. We were in a much stronger position emotionally, and the financial classes we attended put us in a better place financially as well. I was not ignorant to the potential we had for our marriage to crack under the strain. I had made several friends during the previous 15 months who were struggling with infertility as well. Some of their marriages were not fairing as well as ours was. I thanked God for my husband's patience with me and I was grateful God has softened my heart enough to stop pushing my husband away when I needed him. I now desperately clung to "my partner in battle" as we moved forward in our hopes to have a baby. Going back to Dr. Greer was different this time in that we finally acknowledged *together* that we needed more help than what Dr. Hayes could offer. It was a nice feeling to *trust that* my husband was on the same page as me. In late February, we scheduled another consult with Dr. Greer and went in, holding our breath and our pocket books tightly, and prepared for the worst.

Thankfully, Dr. Greer did not require retesting of anything on my husband, and we were able to jump right in, as they say, which was a nice boost to my "instant gratification… proactive… now, now, now" mind-set. The overall conception attempts were much the same as our earlier efforts with on minor difference. Dr. Hayes would still call in the scrip for Clomid and manage the female side of things. We would still track ovulation with the pee sticks from Dr. Hayes' office. These were technically the same thing as drugstore sticks, but somehow much more costly. And finally, instead of doing all the fun stuff at home, Kevin would donate his "contribution" to Dr. Greer's capable on-site lab techs and they would process it for optimal Olympic-level swimmers. After that, Dr. Greer and/or any two of his crew of nurses would do the final installation process for us. This one *minor* tweak in our plans had officially wiped the stork completely out of the picture.

We waited until my next cycle began in early March, did our new math, took our Clomid, and scheduled our necessary appointments with Dr. Greer's office. Around that time seemed like a great time to send an update to my family via e-mail. And so it went:

> Hey guys, it's been awhile since we've sent one of these e-mails to our families, but we're just now finally making some progress. We are officially scheduled to go in for our first round of IUI tomorrow at 11:30. We'll be leaving the house around 10:30 to do all the pre-treatment stuff and should be home around 1:00-ish (give or take). I'm so nervous right now, but also excited. Some people have asked, "What does this do for you?" Essentially, this will boost our chances a full 15 percent (thereby, giving us a 20 percent chance) of conception. There is a tiny risk to me for this procedure, but it's highly unlikely anything would go wrong (and frankly well worth it, given our chances otherwise).
>
> Please take a moment tomorrow and pray for us. We are planning for three to six months of this and hoping/praying/holding our breath that one of them will "stick." Pray for steady hands on the doctors, pray for optimal health for Kevin and I, and pray, pray, pray for babies! If this works, we'll know by the beginning of April. If it does not work, you'll get another one of these messages next month asking for the same stuff. You might as well just get comfortable on your knees 'cause we're likely to need lots of prayer and support in the coming months."

I got the usual round of platitudes and positive thinking remarks from family and a few logistical questions from parents about exact time they could expect a call that I was "okay," but otherwise everyone remained relatively silent.

That first IUI day was a bit nerve-racking for us both I think. Kevin had to do his part on a timetable that was only slightly pressure-induced. We then rushed to the doctor's to turn in his man-sample and wait the appropriate hour of time for them to process things. Finally, they called us back to a room and I proceeded to don the ever-elegant large paper napkin over my now chilly lap and wait. Admittedly, I was very nervous. I had experienced a few "bad apples" by way of gynecological visits in the past and was nervous in general about anything that hurt "down there." This procedure was wholly unknown to me. Sure, they had technically explained the procedure to me, but it did not help me much from a comfort standpoint. From what I could tell at that time, it seemed they were going to insert what looked like a coffee stirrer straw up my wahoo, through the cervix (which I had always considered a one-way exit door until then), and then inject a pink-ish syrup-y fluid filled with my husband's hyped-up swimmers. While it *seemed* like a relatively easy process and was done in the office with no anesthetic of any kind, I was nonetheless terrified. I thought, *Would it hurt? Was that coffee stirrer oversized in any way? Was my cervix freakishly small somehow? Would the pink-ish fluid hurt at all going in, and would it come back out? Is it even supposed to come out? And if it stays in, will my child be born.... pink? How would we know after all that lab processing and time spent that we had actually injected live swimmers and not dead ones?* The questions were non-stop and growing more ridiculous by the minute.

The whole process stressed me out immensely, not including the $350-plus we were then spending on all this. When the good doctor arrived with one of his nurses to do the deed, I was already wound up like a spring. Kevin was there, the whole time, holding my hand like a dutiful husband. We figured if it worked, at least he could say he was in the room when we conceived our child. I laid back, assumed the position (scooting precariously close to falling off the edge of that stupid table), and literally held my breath. Admittedly, it was not that bad. Sure, it was not a pedicure and a latte level of comfort, but it was merely pressure and some mild discomfort that lasted a whopping two seconds, and then the whole thing was over. Voilà! I was officially inseminated by a doctor for the first time ever. I closed my eyes and envisioned my husband and the good doctor taking out their shotguns and blowing a load of buckshot into the stork. Any romance about this time in our life was sufficiently… dead as a doornail!

Dr. Greer and staff left the room and instructed us to lay there for about fifteen to twenty minutes and wait before getting up. After he left, I promptly started to cry and shiver. It was, no doubt, a very physical reaction to all my nerves and worry up to that point. My brave face and well-timed humor was gone and I was laying there, cramping slightly, draped in paper, FREEZING, and feeling very vulnerable.

HEATHER D. NELSON

Kevin was a saint. He leaned over, hugged me, and held my hand. He then proceeded to put his coat over me to help me get warm, and then rubbed my hands and feet to help me relax a bit and even prayed over me that God would let this work for us and protect us through this process. I always felt better when he would pray for me, I do not know why, but his voice in prayer soothed me.

After about five minutes or so, I was much better and we waited the remaining time and then got up and left with instructions to test for pregnancy in exactly two weeks using a home pregnancy test. If it was negative, I would call Dr. Hayes for more Clomid and we would do this all over again. With that, we left; officially artificially inseminated with every chance that we would now start our family. Financially we were on track, our marriage was stronger than ever, our communication skills improved, and even my faith was better than ever. Things were looking way up for us. Then, the two week wait began… again.

The Wait Is On

That particular two-week wait was difficult for me. There were too many things in my mind for me to be able to process any *one* thing all the way through. Not only was this the first official time of trying with, what I then thought was, major medical intervention… but the original due date of Peanut was arriving. That alone was enough to make me cringe a little and want to hide from the world but alas there was more to do. My husband's birthday was the day before Peanut's due date, and my in-laws were in town for a visit to celebrate. As if all of that was not enough to keep my mind reeling a bit, we were still attempting to pry ourselves off the credit card habit we had formed and switch over to a strictly cash basis These lifestyle changes were working, but in truth were still a "work in progress." With all of that hitting at once, I was both glad to keep busy and frustrated at the level of stuff in my way of focusing on what I was *sure* was our guaranteed shot at a baby.

I decided it was best to try and simplify things as much as possible and take one activity at a time. The birthday was low-key, the budget was livable, and my in-laws were pleasant as always. The event, as a whole, was a nice one and my husband always did enjoy more casual events anyways so I felt it was a successful, albeit, calm occasion. Peanut's due date hit me harder than I would have imagined, however. I was surprised that after all that time I even remembered the due date, much less noticed that the day was approaching. A lot of those old feelings came rushing back and I found myself very low-spirited and even a little heartsick. No one said anything other than Kevin, but I think at least my in-laws knew. It was a quiet day that day which suited my heavy heart perfectly. Sadly, all the other events took so much of my time, that by the time we finally took a home pregnancy test that resulted in a big negative, it was almost anti-climatic.

April and May were a repeat of March's attempts, and subsequent failures, at conception. By now, I was up to 150mg doses of Clomid. The drugs were much more intense, and my cycles were becoming more and more painful. Even with all that though, the overall procedure had not changed:

- Call Dr. Hayes and get drugs
- Test at home for ovulation
- Call Dr. Greer and schedule IUI
- Go in, do the deal, wait
- Two weeks later, test for pregnancy
- Get big fat negative—cry and despair
- Spend a week or so eating or drinking whatever I wanted to try and put it out of my mind
- Start period
- Reset my Internal Resolve Gauge
- Lather…rinse…repeat

On paper, those few months of IUI with Dr. Greer might have seemed like a harmless and routine protocol to follow. In fact, I had expected that the repetitive monotony of it all would have allowed me some comfort. However, as my journals of that time would show, there was not even a small modicum of grace or dignity left in me:

Friday, March 28, 2008

I'm noticing today that I'm doing remarkably well considering I'm on Clomid (150mg) and took my second dose last night. I'm really doing well. I did have a hard time waking up (as usual) and my brain is a bit foggy… but I'm excited about the day and not at all irritated or bothered…

Saturday, March 29, 2008–The Very Next Day

I took my third dose of 150mg last night… and I'm furious already. Last night I got mad at a box of crackers… this morning I got mad at my hair (literally), my toilet (do not ask), and my dog. I'm trying to remain calm, but my darling husband can tell. He's doing his best to remain cute and funny and distract me and basically do whatever he can to help make this easier. Man… do I love him! But it's still hard. I try to keep my comments to myself, not react outwardly to the frustrations, etc., but (as a friend of mine says) I cannot hide the big black storm cloud in my eyes when I look at people. What's worse, I'm scheduled to sing on the worship team at church tomorrow. Both services. Which requires rehearsal tonight from 4:00 to 7:00. I really, really do not want to upset or hurt anyone, and I'm afraid I'll react and freak out without meaning to. On the other hand, I feel like if I go and just get into the music, I'll relax and enjoy it. I just need to figure out a way to avoid those pesky "people."

Monday, April 7, 2008

Today is not a good day, and this entire weekend was pretty rough too. I took my Clomid and we are waiting to ovulate we can try IUI again. "Waiting" is the key word here.

Saturday was day fifteen: no ovulation

Sunday was day sixteen:–no ovulation

Today is day seventeen:–no ovulation

I'm freaking totally out. I tried to keep myself distracted this weekend, but this morning I simply lost it. I started to cry and worry and panic. There is only one certified reproductive endocrinologist in the entire state of Idaho, and his first appointment is not until the end of May. we'd lose as much as three months before getting to try anything else if this does not work this time. My regular OB/GYN, who I love, is leaving her practice to teach in June, and I am now afraid that I will not be pregnant before she goes and will have to switch OBs and start all over again with a doctor who will not understand my paranoia. Also, I'm frustrated at my husband, which is not the norm, since he's been unendingly supportive and loving during all this crap. The whole reason this cycle may not work is because my body is building immunity to Clomid. We waited a whole four months (while on Clomid) before starting IUI because he wanted to try natural conception and I wanted to be respectful. I agreed with his decision, but now I'm frustrated and scared and worried and panicking that we've waited too long all around, and I'm immune to Clomid and will have to wait three months to see a specialist and start all this over and precious months will go by and I'll still have no baby!

Monday, April 14, 2008

I'm such a hypocrite! Even though I know—know—in my head that it takes as much as nine days for implantation to happen, and therefore there is no point in testing before then… and even though I have sat on my high horse and encouraged other women to just be patient, remain positive, hopeful, etc., etc., etc. and not obsess and test too early… and even though I myself said that this time would be different, this time I would not obsess and start testing so soon etc., etc, etc… -I cracked. I tested. I peed on a stick and it came back with a big, fat, huge, blaring negative! It's too soon to be sure, I know, but I cannot help but feel that this cycle is another big waste, and that there is something wrong with me that we do not know about yet, and we're just pissing money down the drain each IUI we attempt.

Wednesday, April 30, 2008

Monday evening around five, my primary care physician called and said that my blood pregnancy test was negative. Then Tuesday I woke up feeling like utter crap and had started my period. I was pretty low yesterday… really emotional (not like me) and just generally not feeling well. Headache, crampy, stomach upset… not myself at all. I quit work early and tried to rest and let my darling husband pamper me (after a full-blown emotional melt down that is). I feel very 'spread thin' emotionally and physically and incapable of handling anything. My darling husband is truly an angel. I melted down last night and he handled it great. We did the math and my worst days on Clomid this time will be on our anniversary and my birthday next Wednesday and Thursday. Yikes. But my darling husband is making plans. We're moving up our anniversary to this weekend and my birthday to the weekend after. I love him, I love him, I love him, but even with all that, I'm beside myself with exhaustion…

The good Dr. Greer had told us to expect three to six months of this before "the law of diminishing returns" kicked in, so we had planned accordingly and even had cash to do it all without incurring more debt. That was a small but tangible blessing at the time. Under that miniscule glimmer of positivity though, Kevin and I were both feeling that something was still not working out. Since the miscarriage, we had tried a solid seven months with various levels of Clomid, three of those with IUI, and still had no luck. My cycles were getting more and more uncomfortable and overall, we both felt like that we were spinning our wheels with the approach Dr. Greer and Dr. Hayes had laid out for us. We discussed our thoughts on the matter, and agreed that it was time to do something different. We had gone as far on Clomid as Dr. Hayes would allow, and Dr. Greer could only really help us if we chose to do more IUI's. In the fertility game that meant it was time to go to a reproductive specialist. When we finally decided that our next step was a specialist, my heart skipped a beat and I swear I heard dramatic music swelling in the background. I had already, in my mind, endured so much poking and prodding and pharmaceutically induced insanity. What more would a specialist put me through… and was I really ready for it?

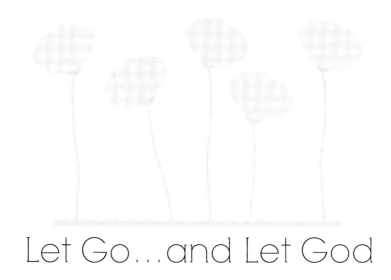

Let Go…and Let God

The month of May marked another turning point in our family planning efforts and in my walk with God. By now, we had turned to the counsel of our associate pastor (Pastor Jeff) in our church. He and his wife were new to our church and in fact had just joined up back when we were recovering from the loss of Peanut. Overtime, we had gotten to know them and learned that they were *great*. We liked them both once we got to know them. Furthermore, they had gotten to know more about us, as a couple, as well as our procreation troubles. With the friendship between the four of us growing, it was a natural leap to ask Pastor Jeff to begin praying for us and counseling us through the coming trials that we were volunteering ourselves for.

So, early in May, we invited Pastor Jeff over and asked that he pray for us. That was scary to me but it was a small enough commitment in the beginning, I felt. I was a little nervous before he arrived because I knew he'd need to ask a few questions and I'd have to put a certain level of trust in him that I had not done yet. I was sure he *could* handle it, but was still unsure *how* he would handle it. I had already, sadly, learned that it was hard to share my infertility status with people. I never knew how they would react and I had experienced some pretty horrendous responses. I prayed that trusting Pastor Jeff with this would be a wise decision.

When Pastor Jeff finally arrived, he spent several *hours* at our kitchen table asking questions, which was unexpected. Not at all the courtesy one or two surface level questions I expected, but rather he engaged us in an in-depth discussion of our predicament. I was surprised, but it turned out to be exactly what we needed, at exactly the time when we needed it. Pastor Jeff spent a good part of the time trying to understand where we were both at spiritually and logistically. He asked the basic questions like, "How long had we been trying?" and, "When was the miscarriage?" He also got into deeper stuff and asked me what treatments were we doing now, what was the financial cost, and what was Kevin's role, etc. He even went so far as to ask us what fears we had about the whole process, which I did not see coming. When he finally started inputting his thoughts, Pastor Jeff immediately put some of my lingering fears to rest that I had been lugging around. Specifically, I had long been struggling with some major spiritual, personal, and marital struggles that I could not reconcile in my mind. It seemed silly after all the huge epiphany moments I had already experienced in the previous year, and yet there was still stuff tagging along in my mind that I could not shake. Things I was too embarrassed or too afraid to ask others about. Things like:

- Was I being unfaithful by pursuing medical specialists to have a baby?
- Was my lack of confidence each month in said specialists a sign of my lack of faith in the power of God?
- Was my husband's abundance of faith a sign that he did not care enough about the process to be as worried and emotionally invested as I was?
- Was I somehow deficient (lazy) because I was overwhelmed and could not seem to handle anything in my regular day-to-day life anymore?

These questions and more had been haunting me off and on for what was now the better part of a year and a half. Pastor Jeff was very quick to put these to bed, finally, in a way that was both loving and finite.

He explained that God created all things, including people who go to medical school and become specialists. God gave these people a desire to seek this knowledge. God also gave these people to the world in order to help us overcome physical ailments and conditions. If God does not want something to work, it simply will not work. Me pursuing these avenues of treatment was not somehow spitting in God's face. In fact, nothing I could do would somehow be beyond God's power. He's GOD. I took a big sigh of relief when Jeff put that fear to rest. Ever since some misguided woman blurted out to me that she felt infertility treatments were just ignorant people playing God, I had been carrying that gigantic questions mark around in my mind. It was awesome to have the confirmation that my fear was just as misguided as that one woman's opinion.

Pastor Jeff went on to explain that my husband's abundance of faith in God did *not* mean he did not care, nor did my lack of faith mean I was somehow deficient in God's eyes. Rather, Kevin had been given a different and unique perspective on the whole situation. Pastor Jeff explained that this unique perspective was a gift from God in that He made Kevin and I different *so* that we could be a team in stressful times. In this way we would not be so similar that stressful times overtook us. I was not lazy or deficient in any way for being overwhelmed. Simply put, I had been beat up for six-plus months and I was entitled to *not* want to do anything. For that matter, it was completely understandable that I would be overwhelmed, and that tied in to the "God gifted us differently" explanation as to why my husband was much more capable at handling life right then than I was. That was how God intended it!

Pastor Jeff was great. He even used a wonderful analogy to explain an important marital truth to my husband and I. He talked about those old-time, seaworthy ships, the kind with the long bow sticking out of the front of the ship. The job of that long bow was to break up ice and water so that the ship could maintain structural integrity and float through the water a lot faster. This would also allow for a smoother ride for the sailors and passengers aboard and ultimately increase safety as well. In the analogy Pastor Jeff gave, our marriage was the ship, my husband was the bow, and our whole family unit was the precious cargo being ferried across the waters of life. God gave my husband and I just the right amount of the faith we needed, when we needed it. We were currently in an unbalanced phase in our lives. I was physically and emotionally drained and had little strength for much else. Kevin, on the other hand, was not put through the physical demands of drugs, tracking, timing, etc., that I was and had more reserves to pull from. As such, this was a time in our marriage for him to be the bow. His job was to be the strong arm in our daily life "breaking the ice" for me. Infertility was the stormy sea in our life, at that time, and I was struggling to keep my head above water. It was Kevin's time to support me and make my daily walk a little easier in whatever way he could. Likewise, it was my time to ride my husband's coattails a bit and let him carry me through this rough patch, or be the safe cargo floating the waves. Pastor Jeff said that this time of Kevin carrying me through was not only appropriate, but also expected considering what we were trying for. It would not be forever and who knows what the future would bring, but for now, *this* is what our marriage needed and *this* is what God had prepared us for.

Pastor Jeff then went on to specifically address my husband directly. He told Kevin that it was his time to step up as a man and take that lead role. He went on to say that God *wants* men to take the lead in a marriage, but that often times men let the wives take on that role because it is easier. Easier for the wife to stay organized and on top of things, and easier for the husband to sit back and let her. But when husbands step up and take the lead role God intended for them, the whole marriage runs smoother. I was secretly giving Pastor Jeff a standing ovation by now. I had so badly wanted Kevin to be that type of leading man in our life and here sat our pastor pretty much telling my husband that very thing. It was a great moment for me... and then that moment was gone as Pastor Jeff directed his gaze at me.

Gulp!

As it turned out, my job was to *let* my husband step up. I sort of chuckled at first at how easy and cool that would be. I would soon realize how hard that was in reality though. That would mean letting go of some of my control and *trusting* my husband to do things as *he* thinks they should be done, not as I think they should be done. That was a tall order for me. Furthermore, I had to literally give my husband permission to tell me "no." As an independent woman raised by a single mother, the concept of giving a man control over me enough to tell me "no" was not something I was prepared to do. But that was what I had to do. Kevin was allowed, ordered by God even, to tell me "no!" No, I could not volunteer for one more project; I was too busy. No, I could not plan one more social activity; I was too tired. And no, I could not try to host, help, support, or anything else; it was time to focus on me. Time to focus on our family. Time to be selfish a little and let him, as the man, call the shots. Not make the calls on just the big stuff, but also little things, like opening and sorting the mail, organizing the bills, even grocery shopping. My internal ovation for Pastor Jeff had ceased and I was now mentally calculating how long it would take for my resolve to crack in my efforts to let Kevin tell me "no."

In the end, though, I was very sure this would never happen... all this great advice. After all, *how many husbands actually work to take that kind of an active role*, I thought? And what are the chances that a formerly controlling, overly organized wife would actually hand the keys to *that* kingdom over willingly? In all truth I was thinking, "*Yeah sure, Pastor Jeff, he'll step up to the lead and I will totally relax and things will not fall apart... you betcha!*" I felt, smugly for sure, that I was safe in my belief that I would never need to *actually* let go since my darling husband would never really *want* to take that much of an active role in the minutia of life that he otherwise loved having me take point on. But much to my surprise, my husband chimed in that he was thrilled to do it. My jaw hit the floor as I listened to Kevin discuss that he knew he needed to step up, but did not know how. Sure, he had done little things, but until I would emotionally breakdown each month, he had no clue how to handle things. I would handle everything until I would finally crack under the strain of another failed cycle and suddenly need DEFCON 1 level pampering and then he would be all to happy to oblige, but until then, he felt his hands were tied. It was not until those moments of overload that I would finally *let* him support me. He told Pastor Jeff that he was glad to finally have a defined role of things he could do to support me and help me through this time on a day-to-day basis. I could not believe how easily Kevin had flipped and was so suddenly willing to take on this change in our roles. I, on the other hand, was a bit harder to change.

It was not easy for me to let my husband step up and say "no" once in awhile but it was a relief at times. With all the stressors in my life, most of my obligations at that time were just that… obligations. Obligations that I felt I had to do out of some weird sense of guilt. Kevin stepping in and telling me, and the world, "no" was sometimes a wonderful treat for me. But the other part was hard for me, the "letting him take the *control* over things and stop worrying about them" part. Geez, that was hard. I mean, worrying has often been known by those who dearly love me as my own personal hobby. At that time, it was a twenty-nine-year-old habit I was not going to easily put down and one I came by quite honestly. In fact, my grandmother's capacity for worry was the stuff of legend, after all. I could claim that I was genetically predisposed to fretting. I had to school myself a bit and trust my husband more in the day-to-day things of our life. Furthermore, I had to accept the gentle reminders from my husband when I would slip up and try to assume that lead role. Talk about a challenge. Sometimes those gentle reminders had to be heard daily!

In the end, Pastor Jeff was absolutely right. By letting go of things more and letting my husband step up into a leadership role in our lives, I was ultimately relieved. I could not imagine how much pressure I had put upon myself with outside obligations that truly were not as important as I had built them up to be. It was not an easy transition to make, but it was needed at the time, and it did so much for my emotional well-being to let go of those nagging questions and lean on my husband more. I had gained yet another way to trust in him in a way I had, really, never truly trusted in him before. And He never let me down. Not once! Sure, he did not do things the way I would have done them at times, and yeah, I may have accomplished some tasks more efficiently than he did, but that was not the point. I was learning that marriage is not a race to see who can be the most organized or have the best time management abilities. Marriage is a partnership, and this was a prime example of a time when one partner needed a little more and the other partner could clearly give it. I had a laugh when I finally let all this sink in. God knew this all along. I thought about all the finance classes and forgiveness epiphanies and I realized then that it was all leading up to this phenomenal lesson. The marriage of ultimate success was intended to be built as the Bible spelled out so plainly. Husbands loving their wives, laying down their own lives, and leading the household, and wives submitting to their husbands and giving trust and respect. *Duh!*

Finally Listening

All these past months, I was stressed and worried and exhausted and emotional and weak and lost and you name it—that was me. I would struggle to keep my head above water, and then breakdown each month when that big, fat, negative pregnancy test would come in. I would wallow in my self-pity for the few precious drug-free days I was allowed and indulge in whatever I could indulge in during that time. Some months it was hot baths and lunch meat, but most months it was a bottle of wine and a chocolate binge. Then the next month, I would bolster up my courage and do it all over again. The cycle was as exhausting to me emotionally as the drugs were to me physically, and the wear and tear of the two on my faith was about more than I could bear.

Kevin, on the other hand, was always rock solid. He was forever confident that God would provide and never yielded that we could do this if we waited, tried, prayed, planned, etc. He would always tell me, "Let the doctors worry about the medicine and let me worry about the money, you just worry about relaxing." Part of me knew things would be much easier if I would just listen to my husband's repetitive advice. But I didn't…I continued to fret each and every day for the entire time between the miscarriage and our current cycles. God had sent me exactly what I needed, in my husband, and I missed it over and over and over again. I was wrapped up in my struggle, trying to plan, chart, organize, steer, finance, *control* or whatever my way to a baby, that I had failed to see the pillar of strength that my husband had continued to be. Not only was this bad for my faith in God, but it was not that great for my faith in my husband either. I couldn't help but wonder how many times I wished he would pick up the slack and do a little more or worry more like me just so I would know he cared? In reality, he did care and he *wanted* to pick up the slack, he only needed me to finally let it go. When I did, the results were glorious. I was able to trust and lean on him in a fabulous new way. In turn he, as a husband, felt far more involved and useful in our process than before. All in all, that little visit with Pastor Jeff was a God-send!

We ended that day with prayer and a promise from Pastor Jeff to check in on us periodically as we moved forward with our plans to visit the reproductive endocrinologist. With that done, we trudged forward to our June 6, 2008 appointment, ready to take on the world. We had a new plan of how to handle the world at-large, and we felt more capable of handling whatever the new doctor might have in store for us. I was once again recharged and felt good about our path. I was nervous about letting Pastor Jeff into our little world of infertility madness. I was unsure how he would handle the awkward and personal details of our struggle, much less how he would address the faith versus science dilemmas I was struggling with. After he had gone, I knew we had made a good choice in allies with him and his wife. At the very least, we had gained much more in prayer and support than we had beforehand. My confidence that our plans were sure to succeed was overflowing. I just knew that with all our life lessons learned and safely tucked away, it was now time for us to have a family. Surely it would be safe to dust off some of those old "due date" dreams, right?!

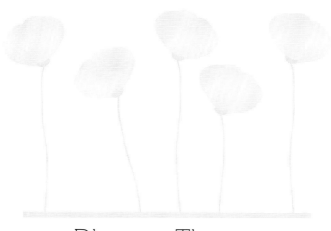

Phase Three

The days leading up to our first appointment with the new doctor, Dr. Slater, were nerve-racking for me. It was another huge leap to finally jump to a doctor who specialized in reproductive medicine. That gave me great hope that we would finally get some answers as to what all had been going on in the previous year. I imagined finally getting answers to why I miscarried, why I could not get pregnant again, what were the better treatment plans for Kevin's swimmers, and more. I had such hope. But the flip side of that was a whale-sized amount of fear to match. There was only one reproductive medicine office in the entire state, what would I do if they did not like me? For that matter, what if the doctor and me do not get along and I do not like the way they choose to approach our issues? What if they tell me there is nothing they can do for me, or what if they told me that my options were slim I should spend a fortune on IVF or adoption and otherwise quit trying? What if they looked at my chart and literally laughed me out of the office for trying to even waste their time?! For every hope-filled thought I clung to, a worry snuck in right behind it, and the end result was my growing anxiety being banged back and forth like a tether ball. By the time the day came for our first visit, I can honestly say I was wound up like a spring... again.

Yet More Doctors

The day of the appointment was, well, not at all like I expected. I knew that Dr. Slater was female, was rated one of the best specialists in the Northwest, and was highly recommended to me by three different doctors, but otherwise I had no idea what to expect. I was very nervous, overall, but I imagined her being a lot like Dr. Hayes: educated, knowledgeable, but loving and soft like a big sister who is easy to talk to and understands when you cry your way through a question. I expected the office to be filled with women nurses who would love on you all the time and share your pain and worries with you, and it would feel like a big reproductive sorority of some kind. I even had some crazy notion that there would be some kind of fertility-sisterhood secret handshakes and Ya-Ya hats. In otherwords I think I expected the entire clinic to feel like a giant group of friends who would somehow help us HUG our way to a baby.

When we arrived, the waiting room was clean and comfy but plainly decorated and understated. Not the ultra-feminine touch I expected. We did not wait long before they took us back to Dr. Slater's office and we waited in there for her. As we sat, I noticed her office was tasteful but also sparsely decorated. She did have pictures of her and her children and a few key pieces of things that I envisioned were gifts from patients. When she arrived, she was friendly and smiling, she shook both our hands. She was a tiny petite little woman and I had to stifle a chuckle when she sat down behind her giant desk in her enormous chair and immediately whipped out a super thick file. She spent the first few minutes reviewing my gargantuan medical and reproductive history, as was sent over by the small squadron of doctors we had already seen. I remember actually blushing when I saw how thick my file was. Surely, I thought, my file being this thick could send her the wrong message that we were somehow going to be difficult patients. Dr. Slater didn't seem to notice at all though as she thumbed through each and every page reviewing and taking notes. She asked

HEATHER D. NELSON

pointed questions to things that were a bit vague in the records, but kept it all very clinical and business-like. Almost as if she was just a doctor and not my sorority sister. I was not expecting this semi-cold approach and it caught me off guard. Being a bit thrown in the beginning turned out to be good though since I did not cry through the whole appointment. I stared and answered questions as instructed, as if I were that kid in the principle's office. After all the Q&A, she laid out the basics that you always learn about in high school health class but take for granted in your adult years.

What do you need to make a baby? Eggs and sperm. If you want to make a baby the old-fashioned way, you also need fallopian tubes and a uterus. She then explained how we already knew about certain pieces of this overly simplistic puzzle, but not all. We knew I ovulated and had ovaries. After all, I had gotten pregnant at least once, and though I needed Clomid to kick-start the process, it was clearly possible to get me to ovulate again. We also knew that we had sperm, since we had all the analysis done with Dr. Greer and seen exactly what quality and quantity of swimmers we were dealing with. After those two key pieces what was left was the fallopian tubes and my uterus. Peanut survived long enough to prove that I had them both at some point, but something was clearly amiss and there was potential I no longer had functioning tubes or even a viable uterus. This was a surprise to me to say the least. It had not occurred to me, prior to that appointment, that I might not have a viable uterus. And if that was true… does that mean my somehow "unviable" uterus is what killed Peanut? The questions in my mind were compounding and stifling. As much as I was struck speechless by the thought of an unviable uterus, I managed to ask the one obvious question to Dr. Slater at this point: "How do we find out if my tubes and uterus are okay?" Dr. Slater told us of a very simple and common procedure called a Hysterosalpingogram (HSG). They would inject dye into my uterus and look to see if it was open and clear in my tubes, etc. She went on to say that the whole process would take ten minutes, be relatively painless, and give us quick answers on the final pieces of the puzzle. It was one of the few diagnostic tests we had not had run that she insisted we do before moving forward. I inwardly snickered at how much the medical community liked to describe vaginal procedures of any kind as "relatively painless." The idea of injecting DYE up into my uterus and through my fallopian tubes sounded anything but "relatively painless."

Kevin and I agreed the HSG was a smart choice and we scheduled that for the following Monday. We then jumped into the "here are your options" portion of the meeting. Up until now, we had experienced one pregnancy without IUI, but 7 failed cycles with Clomid and three of those also included IUI's. Dr. Slater pointed out that the one other thing we never really had during all this time was any kind of real follicle monitoring to see how my ovaries responded or if I did indeed ovulate. With that knowledge, Dr. Slater left the choice in our hands. If we wanted to pursue more aggressive IUIs with injectable drugs and close ovulatory monitoring, she would approve and support that for us. It would increase our chances and be a cheaper step than IVF. On the other hand, since we had already been trying for so long, if we wanted to jump straight into IVF and avoid anymore IUIs, she would approve and support that as well. She gave a case for each and then leaned back in her big office chair and let us decide. IVF was always looming in our minds and we had already discussed that to some degree prior to this meeting. We both agreed that we were not ready for IVF yet (both financially and emotionally). Kevin and I both wanted to continue to try the IUI option, but with closer monitoring and injectable drugs to ensure we were getting good responses. It would be more intense, but we would at least have much better assurance if it was working. I had expected her to push IVF more, but she was very gracious and respectful of our choice. Dr. Slater then told us the best news we had heard in months. Most healthy couples who have optimum rates only have a 25–30 percent chance to get pregnant each month. That decreases with age, complications, etc., and we already knew we were down in the 5 percent range ourselves. She felt confident that if we could get me to ovulate, she could put us right back up there in the 25–30 percent range like everyone else. Even with Kevin's morphology issues, she was not at all worried and felt good about our chances. I'm pretty sure the heaven's opened up and I could actually hear the hallelujah chorus right then. I could have climbed over her big giant desk and shoved that behemoth file out of the way and hugged her petite little neck at this point. Up until now, we had gotten the standard clinical stats response from all doctors, and no promises or guarantees of any kind. In fact, the most positive response of any kind had been some phrase that involved "the law of diminishing returns." To have a specialist flat out say that she was confident she could get us pregnant was bliss. It was like rainbows, fluffy kittens, chocolate, and spa days all wrapped up in one silver-lined billowy cloud of goodness.

In the meantime, she continued, since I was on cycle day six and already in the office, Dr. Slater decided a pelvic exam was in order, as well as an ultrasound and complete blood work on both me and Kevin to save us a trip and some office visit fees. She said that if things looked good, we could start a cycle *that day*. I thought, *finally, my instant gratification itch is going to be scratched.* She then led us out of her office to our various rooms and we began. My mind was reeling at how quick this was moving forward, and I *knew* that it was a sign from God that we had been faithful and obedient, and would now receive our most sought after reward. I was calculating the due dates in my mind and since we were at specialist office I even threw in a set of dreamed up twins to go with my little fantasy. One boy and one girl of course!

After the nurses took all our blood, the exam came around complete with that *lovely* ultrasound probe. All in all, things looked good. My ovarian follicles were mature and growing and my uterine lining was thick. With that established, Dr. Slater agreed that, barring any complications in the HSG on Monday, we could begin a protocol of injections right away and this could save us another few visits and some money as well. I was practically giddy with excitement and in the far back of my mind, I was dreaming of maternity clothes and baby showers again. She explained all about the various drugs and injections, but overall, it was a simple process. The protocol looked roughly like this:

- Start Clomid the same time for five days
- Begin Menopur injections for two days
- Have ultrasound on Friday to see if I'm ready to trigger

- Trigger shot when ready, then IUI
- Two weeks later, come in for bloodwork to confirm pregnancy status

They gave us a crash course on how to do the injections (which my husband dutifully took notes and stepped up to be my official injection man) and then instructions on how to get the drugs. Turns out they had a handy mail order pharmacy that they used that would send the drugs right to our door, including needles, sharps container, and more. It was a pre-setup process and made things really simplistic.

I left that appointment with a completely renewed spirit. I was surprised and relieved at how efficient and business-like Dr. Slater was. I was thrilled to have a mail order pharmacy ship what I needed to my house without any guess work. I was utterly giddy at the prospect that I no longer had to track my BBT, or use home ovulation kits, or even home pregnancy tests. The doctor would monitor all that for me, and all I had to do was pop a few pills, take a few injections, and otherwise sit back and follow instructions. I walked out of that appointment with a folder full of info, four prescription slips for the pharmacy, an HSG scheduled for three days from then, an ultrasound scheduled for a week out, and a mail order shipment of injectable drugs on the way to my house. It was overwhelming and scary, but I was psyched to finally feel like I was going to get somewhere in this struggle. *We were finally moving forward!* When Monday arrived, the HSG went off without a hitch and the radiologist who was doing the procedure seemed positive that all looked well. So that was it. We had eggs, we had sperm, we had tubes, and a uterus. Hooray for sperm and a uterus! All we needed now was a little arithmetic to put it all together into a baby! Our prayers were uplifting at this point and full of hope. We knew our time had come and God would finally give us *our* baby.

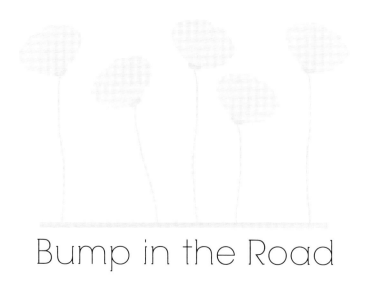

Bump in the Road

The following week, I had taken my Clomid and I am fairly sure I floated through the side effects riding simply on the high of knowing our time was finally coming. I was super thrilled when the drugs arrived at our house, and when the day came to start the injections I was almost—no wait, not almost—I *was* excited about it. I could not wait to finally stick myself with that needle and feel like I was taking a step toward motherhood. I envisioned it in my mind and it was perfect. Sure, we had struggles, but now with all these drugs, we'd have *twins*, and all the struggles would be worth it to look at our beautiful family! And yes, *one boy* and *one girl*... hello? I was flitting through my days when the phone rang, and all my good delusions came to a screeching, grinding, crumbling halt.

I had finally started to learn that when the doctor calls you themselves (not a nurse or some other underling), it is a bad sign. So when my phone rang and Dr. Slater's voice was on the other end, my heart skipped a beat or two. Apparently, the radiologist who said things looked good was not entirely accurate: there was a "mass" in my uterus. Dr. Slater described it as scar tissue, most likely left over from my miscarriage. She explained that the problem was not so much the scar tissue itself, but the amount and position of it. It was smack dab in the middle of my uterus and it covered over one-third of the total surface area. In short, I could not have gotten pregnant under just about *any* circumstances, and if I did, the fetus would not likely survive long since all that scar tissue would affect my uterine environment and the ability for a baby to implant. All my pretty fantasies began to float away and in my desperate attempt to hold on to them, I actually tried to argue with the doctor at this point. I did not care that she had mega-dollars and years worth of education and training under her belt. Surely I could enlighten her and get her to change her mind.

I told her that the nice radiologist man said it was nothing and that all looked good. Dr. Slater was gracious and agreed that my tubes were clear and wonderful, but that this mass of scar tissue simply had to come out. She also explained that this was likely the reason that all my cycles since the miscarriage had been painful and crampy She even seemed nearly convinced it was the sole reason we had not conceived again by now. I was utterly deflated when I said, "well fine, I have to have the scar tissue out… now what?" According to Dr. Slater, the earliest they could schedule me for was another week, and I would have to stop all fertility meds and instead go on birth control pills to elongate my cycle and stop my period for the procedure. So for me that meant that after being hyped-up on Clomid for a week, I would have to turn around and take birth control pills. I knew I was not prepared mentally for that kind of hormonal slingshot.

Shifting Gears

Needless to say, I was discouraged at this point. After having such a positive and forward-moving appointment the previous week, and after having already started a new round of drugs and having hope that we had a chance, I was completely slammed by the news that there was yet another thing wrong with my wretched body. Kevin was all on board to hold off on our cycle again and get me healthy, as usual, but I was thinking that maybe God was punishing me again. Maybe all this scar tissue was remnants from my hard lived party days when I was younger, and it was now creeping back in on me. I became deeply afraid at this point as well that maybe this is why we lost Peanut to begin with. I had always held out some kind of hope that we would be okay, but this was another blow to my thinking that maybe we would have a baby one day. I began to envision my shallow shell of a life with no children in it. I feared I would become that old woman filling the void with a small herd of pets. I could see me sitting around church as a senior citizen, surrounded by fellow blue-haired jewels all chatting up their grandchild's latest accomplishment, and me, with pictures of my cats wearing funny hats. As a woman, I would forever be a shallow excuse of an otherwise fulfilled life. My existence would no longer be as the caretaker of the next generation, but rather as a selfish ode to myself. And when the golden years came, and my husband was called home to the Lord, I would be that little old lady in a nursing home with no visitors who chats to all the orderlies about my magazine collection. And this scar tissue—this undefinable "mass" that made my uterus unviable–would follow me throughout my days as a constant reminder of how I had squandered my good health with my sinful nature and thus earned my barren status.

I could just begin to see the inscription on my headstone. It would read *RIP Heather, the poor dear sinned her way into a cattery and died alone.*

The doctor was confident the scarring was from the miscarriage being physically strenuous, and Kevin was very quick to interject that God does not go around randomly punishing people for past sins out of spite. I tried to put those fears to rest *again*, and decided it was time for another e-mail to family:

> Hey guys…well, as you all probably know by now, we were unsuccessful on our third try at IUI, so we went to see the specialist last Friday. She was very experienced and thorough, and we are encouraged that we're in the right hands. One of the things she scheduled was a special test to ensure that my " equipment " was all functioning properly with no blockages, etc. It was the only thing we have not had checked on me yet, so the test was on Monday and we got the results yesterday. My tubes looked great, but there is a good amount of scar tissue in my uterus, most likely from the miscarriage. It's explaining a lot

of my pain/discomfort that I've had, but moreover, it's blocking implantation and is almost definitely the reason we've been wholly unsuccessful getting pregnant this past eight months. So, what does this mean? Well, we gotta get it out.

It's a minor day-surgery, and I should be back up and running within a few days. We'll definitely hold off our family planning efforts for several weeks for recovery, but the surgery itself is minor and should be relatively easy. I just got the call and we're scheduled for next Thursday, the nineteenth at 7:00 a.m., so I wanted to give you guys a heads up. We're relieved to finally have some answers, and we're glad that our new doctor is being thorough and proactive about this. It's not even been a week since we first met her and already so much has happened. If this goes as well as we hope, then my pain should be gone and our first one or two attempts after surgery could be successful. Here's hoping! Thanks a million for everyone's prayers and words of encouragement. This has been a difficult and unique journey for us up until now, and we surely appreciate the support of our family during all this. If any of you have questions or want to ask me anything, fire away… we're ready to chat it up!

When the actual day of the surgery arrived, I was scared. Scared of the unknown, scared of the pain, scared of being put under, in general, just plain scared. We showed up on schedule and they immediately took me back and had me take a pregnancy test, you know… just in case. I laughed at how stupid that was, but part of me held my breath and hoped too. But no, negative again. Stupid unviable uterus! I then stripped down and donned the ever-fashionable giant bedsheet, held together with a glorified shoestring and super cool shower cap. They had the anesthesiologist come in and set up my IVs, and he asked how I was doing. I was very honest and told him that I was growing increasingly anxious, to which he replied, "Oh, we'll take care of that." He promptly injected a little bit of happy into my IV. I do not know what it was actually called, but at that point I was calling it "liquid happy." *That* was nice. After that, things were better. They let my husband stay with me in the pre-op room as they asked their other questions. I informed them that I tend to be emotional when I come out from under anesthesia, which they made a note of, but said was a very common reaction. Finally, they wheeled me back to the surgery room. The last thing I recall was being hoisted to another table and having my legs strapped into giant holster-looking things that were padded with that stuff that you see on top of mattresses. I laughed in my mind at how silly my legs looked wrapped in foam egg carton stuff. I wondered who would be the lucky person that had to drag my unconscious butt to the end of the table as I went swiftly into la-la land.

The next thing I knew, I was in recovery and the surgery was done. I was instantly weepy and asked for my husband, so they let him come right back with me as the doctor came over and talked with us both about how things went. She said that all in all, things went very well. They got all the scar tissue out (she even showed us pictures… *ew*) and it all looked good to her. She explained the stint they inserted in my uterus and she gave my husband a slew of instructions on meds and post-surgery protocol. I was gratefully still in la-la land and going in and out of sleep. Kevin took lots of notes, prescription slips, pictures… *ew*, etc., from the doctors and proceeded to call all of my family to let them know I was fine, and then sat there with me the whole time until I was ready to leave and go home. He was an angel and I loved him so much for being there when I was out of it. I will admit to being very uncomfortable, but more relieved that this was over. The doctor even left us with some more positive news. She said that once my new cycle started, we could immediately begin our new protocol we had planned. She even said that we had really good chances in the following two to three months of trying, and that she was going to work really hard to get us pregnant in that time. That thought alone made me feel like all this was worth it. Surely, I thought, I had done all that needed to be done and I could *freaking* get pregnant already!

Recovery from the surgery was pretty much as you would expect. While the stint was still in, I had lots of crampy, uncomfortable pressure and was not good for much of anything short of laying in the recliner with my feet up. I had to take Estrogen pills to speed up my uterus' healing process and I mentally wondered what one more hormone would do to my poor body. My darling husband did typically well in caring for me during those two or three days. Having the stint removed was akin to having a small balloon yanked out of your cervix. I was not graceful about that part at all, but I felt *much* better and was able to move around more. The healing went relatively fast, and I was actually looking forward to being able to chill for awhile and wait for my cycle to start. In fact, I journaled about my relief at having a forced "break:"

Journal Entry
   Well, my darling husband and I have decided to make the most of this forced delay in our baby-making efforts.
   Clearly we will not be triggering, or attempting conception, anytime this month and in fact are anti-trying to conceive until the next four to six weeks is past. So, while I'm nervous about the surgery and recovery, we've decided to live it up a bit.
   Drink wine if we want
   Eat lunch meat every day
   Eat junk food if I feel like it
   Sit in a hot tub
   Have sex strictly for the recreational value!
   I'm a wild woman! I'm hoping to have fun simply being with my husband without the *trying to conceive* stress for a few weeks so that we can "hop on the good foot and do the bad thing" again when the doctor gives us a thumbs up! Too bad we cannot make a weekend getaway or something in the process... that would be really nice!

After all the hassles and stress of going from drug to drug to drug, it was a nice reprieve to have some time to rest and rejuvenate again. Granted, it was a whopping two week reprieve and we jumped right back in, but it was a great two weeks that I needed. During this time, I prayed to God to heal my body *wholly* and not let the scar tissue return. I further asked that He make the coming months fruitful for us and give us, again, *our* baby.

HEATHER D. NELSON

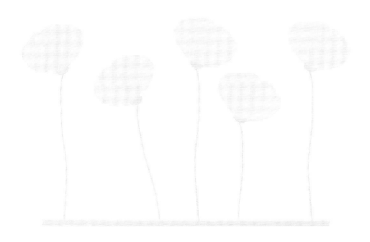

Jumping in with Both Feet

When my next cycle finally started, we began what would be our life for the next several months. To say that I was unprepared for what awaited me would be a grave understatement. I mistakenly thought Clomid prepared me for what to expect. I expected the drugs to make me feel a bit "off" from the norm, but otherwise it would be livable. I was horribly, mistaken. I was a misguided idiot for thinking that what I had undergone up to that point would in *any way* compare to what I was about to go through.

My next cycle began on July 3 and I went in for my first baseline. Baseline is a fancy word they use that basically means they draw blood to check your estrogen levels, and they do a very involved internal "wand" sonogram to check your uterine lining, follicle growth, ovary position, etc. The wand and I, I would soon find out, would become intimately familiar with each other in the coming months, and not always in pleasant terms. The results of all these things would either, pass or fail me to begin a cycle of drugs and injections. If my estrogen level was too high, it could indicate a cyst and we would have to wait out a cycle before trying again. If my uterine lining was too thin, it could require additional drugs for the cycle, but if my ovaries are enlarged or cycling ahead of schedule, the entire thing could be called off and we'd be at square one again. The potential for pitfalls each month was daunting. We also had to do a quick water sonogram to confirm that the scarring was indeed gone and had not grown back. In very non-technical fertility terms, the plumbing was open and we got the thumbs-up to finally move forward. Lucky for me that at this point in the game, I was happy to be able to finally start something and thrilled to hear that all looked good, *finally*. I was excited once again. We had a good and aggressive medical team, a confirmed clean and open uterus ready for a baby, and spectacularly good odds. I felt confident that this would be a short-lived stint and a breeze to go through. Stupid Stupid Stupid Stupid.

My first protocol looked a little like this:

- 100mg Clomid on cycle days three through seven
- Two amp injections of Menopur thereafter until trigger shot (anywhere from 3 to 7 days worth)
- Multiple wand sonograms to monitor follicle growth and uterine lining
- Trigger shot to force ovulation at the determined optimum time
- IUI as planned
- Vaginal Progesterone supplements for two weeks until a beta

All in all, this seemed like a piece of cake to me. However, the effects and stress of all this were slightly delayed, and I had no clue what to expect. Clomid was pretty standard and because I was so uplifted already, I did not notice as many of the nasty moods as I had had before. The injections, though scary to take at first, were not painful at all and my husband even helped me to take them each night because I was a sissy wuss-bag and could not stick myself. I had little to no physical side effects that month other than hot flashes and feeling like my ovaries were the size of bowling balls, but that was to be expected. Prior to all this, I didn't even know I could feel my ovaries and now I was intimately familiar with their location… and size too for that matter.

To my surprise, we had good follicle response with two to three good sized eggs ready for fertilization. In fact, at one of my "wand appointments" I was told that the hardest part of getting a PCOS patient pregnant was getting them to ovulate. .and the rest was easy. And since I was ovulating, the rest should be a piece of cake for me. Who knew I would get cake! I was able to disregard the feeling of being a giant human chicken when the sonographer described how large my many eggs were. The IUI itself was much like before, and the wand monitoring and sonograms in between were a nice reassurance that things were working. Bear in mind though, the wand's comfort level was solely related to whoever was steering in the ramrod that day. After the insemination, I started the progesterone and we began another two-week wait. Of course, by now we called this waiting period the fourteen day descent into madness, but who could blame us after the sheer number of these little fourteen day waits we had already endured. That first cycle was certainly the easiest from a physical standpoint. I was tired, but hopeful, and tired quickly took a backseat to being excited. The end of the two-week wait, specifically the last day, was when the effects of the previous two months (no wait, *years*) kicked into gear.

F.U.B.A.R. Friday

To this day, my husband and I will admit that one of the worst fights we ever had was on a day that we forever will call "F.U.B.A.R. Friday." I will grant you that it is not the most graceful or virtuous name, but that is what we called that day nonetheless. It was a day that will live in marital infamy for us after the havoc that infertility had wreaked on my mind and body. The last few days of the two-week wait were really hard physically. I had thought that my fatigue would go away when I went off the shots, but I was wrong. The progesterone supplements had their hand in things too, and created more fatigue and some other lovely physical discomforts like mild constipation, icky ecosystem feelings, and more. Not to mention, they were just really, really, really incontrovertibly slimy and gross. Beyond all that, the trigger shot manufacturer failed to post a neon-colored warning label that said something to the effect of, "Hey idiot, you're injecting yourself with a ten thousand unit dose of the pregnancy hormone to trigger ovulation… of course you will feel pregnant until it is out of your system—DUH!" So after that first week of the wait, and all my crazy fatigue, I had fully and completely psyched myself up that we were pregnant already. Who could blame me? I was tired, constipated, nauseated, had sore boobs, headaches, the works. Not only that, but I was envisioning my due date and babies (and yes, I envisioned twins again) and wondered how wonderful it would be that our new due date would be the same as Peanut's original due date, and maybe that meant something special as if we had been sent these two new babies to help us heal from Peanut's loss. In other words, I had jumped straight to the finish line in my mind and was waiting for the judges to give me my trophy. God, however, clearly had other plans.

That Friday, as I drove into the office for my very first beta (blood drawn pregnancy test), my father was hundreds of miles away undergoing surgery to amputate part of his toe and repair a severely clogged carotid artery. His health was not good and I hated that I was not there to support him and my stepmother. My brothers were there however, and my family understood that we could not throw all this time and money away on such short notice. I still felt like a selfish heel for not being there and I briefly prayed for my father to come through surgery safely. Of course, I also imagined what it would be like as he called me from recovery and I could tell him we had babies on the way for him. I drove into the office for my pregnancy test, praying the whole time, and waiting for the phone to ring and tell me my daddy was okay. When the nurse called my name in the waiting room, I am certain I leapt off the waiting room chair as if it were on fire. I was spectacularly anxious and keyed up. The nurse drawing my blood asked how I was feeling and I smiled as I said, "Exhausted," to which she replied all too quickly that it was likely *just* the progesterone. I was thinking to myself that this woman must have been a ray of sunshine and happiness to everyone around her.

Despite the nurses "kill-joy" response to my exhaustion, my feelings of surety were not waivered, and I was convinced I was merely a blood test away from being a mommy. Unfortunately, I was told it would take a few hours to find out, so I just drove home and proceeded to wait anxiously by the phone now for both my blood test and an update on my dad. I did not have to wait long. On my way back home to wait for my results, I got a call from Mississippi that the routine surgery my father was having had backfired and things were not going well. He had some complications, as yet unknown, on the operating room table and my family would call me with more information when they had it. I felt bad about not being in Mississippi with my dad already which made this an even harder phone call for me. My brothers reassured me that dad would likely be fine, but they did not have more to tell me yet. I was worried still, but truth be told, I too figured my dad would be fine. I tried to not worry too much and said a little extra prayer to God to please watch over my father. Then I ended that benevolent prayer with, "Oh yeah, and God please, please, please let me be pregnant." After all, that third and fourth "please" was sure to do the trick.

By the time I got home, the young kid that was mowing our lawn that summer called and wanted to come down and do the work that day. Since Kevin and I both worked from home, I said that was fine. Little did I know that such a small mundane task would be the catalyst for a record breaking argument between my husband and I. As the day progressed, I was glued to my cell phone waiting anxiously on my first beta results and instead the phone rings and it is my family again. Dad was wheeled into recovery, but then had to be taken back into the operating room again due to something, as yet unknown, going wrong; they never even saw him in recovery. They would call again and let me know when they knew more, but at this point things were getting worrisome for sure. For either one of my typically stoic brothers to admit they were worried was significant for me and my own levels of panic began to rise. As I hung up the phone I prayed again for my dad to be okay and, of course, for the positive pregnancy results to come quickly. I tried to update my husband on things with my dad but my plans unraveled. He was on an intense phone call for work and was unavailable to chat. As I stood in the door to his office waiting for his call to end, the lawn mowing kid arrived. I hit the mental pause button on that update and instead got the yard work started. As I jumped from one task to another my world became increasingly myopic with anxiety. I was trying too hard to muscle through my day with work and the lawn, and each time I would complete one small benign task, another would take up my field of vision. I never got around to telling my husband about my dad and each time the phone rang, I would jump out of my skin. The hormones and drugs were not helping me cope with this day either.

I attempted to go downstairs and update my husband on what all was going on *again*, but he was in his own world of stress over his new job. AGAIN. He had taken a huge work risk to accept this new position, which was a big transition for him and for us financially, and he seemed buried in that moment with worries that he had somehow screwed up. As such, I could tell I was a little "on my own." This did not sit well with me. I was anxious about the pregnancy test, exhausted and strung out from the drugs, irritated at Kevin's uncharacteristically nonchalant attitude on things, and *intensely* worried about my father. All the while stressing over when the fertility clinic would call with my beta results to assuage my guilt about my not being in Mississippi to begin with. How wonderful would it be to tell my dad that he's going to be a grandfather again. Surely no one would be upset about me missing this surgery if I were actually pregnant now.

About that time, I looked out the window and saw it. Bigger than daylight. There was a huge wasp nest on the fence in our backyard and everything in my world seemed to stop as I visually honed in on it. At that moment, I went from guilt-ridden and worried, straight to angry. You see, the wasp nest on our fence had been there for about two weeks. I had mentioned to my husband several times that he needed to take care of it and he always dismissed it that he would do it later. That morning, before the lawn mowing kid arrived at our house, I mentioned it again to my husband and he blew it off and said that he'd take care of it later. So when I looked out my window after getting the second, or possibly third, disturbing phone call about my father and still no call on the beta, I was more than worried about a whole load of things that I could not control. All that worry and fear and anxiety swiftly channeled themselves into the one part of my life I could tangibly effect: *the bleeping wasp nest.* I saw our poor lawn mower getting obliviously close to the nest as I was opening the door to warn him. Unfortunately, he mowed right past it and got nailed twice, squarely in the forehead, by two big, fat, red wasps. Any other day, this would not have been a crisis, but this day I about snapped. I said a silent seething "*I told you so* " in my head before the panic-stricken and now screaming twelve-year-old kid came flailing into my kitchen. This poor boy unraveled at my kitchen table. Wasp stings hurt, and these were scary big red ones. They were in his face no less, and he had never been stung before, so he was doubly scared. He cried and panicked, and made the *passing* comment between heaving tears that he could not breathe and might be allergic. At that moment, the situation was simply more than I could take.

To my credit, I was the pillar of calm on the exterior. I got some ice from the freezer to put on his head and cool him off, got him sipping some ice water to again cool him off and help him slow his panicked breathing down, and heck, I even remembered that old childhood remedy of baking soda and water to take some of the sting out, which I put on his head. I was slightly impressed with my cucumber-like demeanor. My husband, finally hearing the commotion in his office, came out to check on what was going on. I gave my most lethal glare at him over the boy's head, and said in my most calm and level voice that he had been stung in the face by a wasp *twice.* I have no memory if Kevin said anything at this point. Not that it would have mattered, I was already nailing that coffin shut in my mind…he was toast!

Obviously, the boy did not want to finish the mowing job, so we called his mother who came to get him, and we offered to drive home his lawn equipment for them as well. On our way to his house, I got the call that my dad had thrown a blood clot or *something* that hit his brain and they did not know what the damage was yet since they couldn't get him off the ventilator. I was gasping at the visual of my father on a ventilator but I didn't even have time to react, or even update Kevin, since we were pulling up to our poor lawn kid's house. I stoically hung up the phone, and we unloaded the lawn equipment and got back into our car. In my mind, I was loading my arguments up like buckshot. I was getting ready to shoot my husband down for any multitude of things at that point. After all, our lawn was half cut, the kid was utterly freaked out, I felt horrible that he was stung at *our house*. As far as I was concerned, that was ALL my husband's fault. I was ten shades of furious at my husband for not taking care of that stupid thing weeks ago. Stoking the fires of all my anger was the heaping guilt I was piling on myself over my dad. He was possibly dying and I was the lowest of creatures on earth for not being with him and with my family and that somehow was also my husband's fault. And then,... at that sublime moment of universal perfection,... I got the call from my doctor's office that my beta was negative. Not only negative, but a hormone level in my blood of less than *one*, which is like way, way, way negative. As I hung up the phone, I literally clicked over to the other line as another call came in about my dad. My daddy was still on a ventilator and now would not wake up. They would call again when they knew more.

At that point, I snapped. Truly snapped. I could even hear the proverbial snapping sound in my mind as I lit into my husband with both barrels blazing about the one part of my day that I could tangibly wrap my hands around and throttle at that moment. *The wasp nest*. I railed at him about the irresponsibility of not handling the nest when I first told him to. I blamed him solely for our poor lawn mowing kids panic attack and I think I might have led him to believe we were in law suit danger from it. I am really not sure what all I threw at my poor husband. He, in turn, fired right back at me about his work that day and how stressed he was and that he "did not need this" right then, and a bunch of other stuff I largely ignored. That very short but very hot argument ended with me storming off to the hardware store for wasp killer and him huffing back into his office to work. Nothing was resolved, nothing was even really discussed, but it was the most angry we had mutually been at each other *ever* in the history of our marriage. He was oblivious to what was going on inside of me because I had not verbalized any of it, and I was wholly unaware of what he was dealing with at work because he had not verbalized any of it either. The end result was two normally loving people raging at each other for the insensitivities we had perceived. As I stormed through the hardware store buying wasp repellant, I kept getting updates on dad, about how bad things were. My guilt was suffocating and my frustration at my husband for not being more supportive was brimming to the top of it all. I felt like a human pressure cooker at this point and I just knew if one more thing happened I would explode.

When I got home, Kevin tried to "fix it" by taking the wasp killer from me and handling the nest. Boom! I venomously glared at him and jerked the bottle back out of his hand and screamed, "Oh, no you don't, if you can't set aside your precious work to handle this for the past two weeks, much less deal with the sting issues today any better, you better not *now* decide you can handle things since I've done all the work already. Get back to your office and *I will handle this on my own*!" Of course, he handled my dare equally well by muttering, "Okay," and walking back into his office and *actually* letting me handle the nests. I was furious that he did what I asked and just turned and walked away.

In truth though, I could have cared less about that stupid wasp nest. I know now that this was infertility truly rearing its ugly head. Not only had it begun taking over my life (no money to travel to Mississippi, no way to skip the cycle once started, etc.), but the physical and emotional toll of the drugs had given me very little capacity to handle the *rest* of our life. Day-to-day things were far more daunting to me due to fatigue and emotional wear and tear, but at the time, I did not realize it. I was exhausted and in pain from the drugs, I was overwhelmed at how fast everything had happened, I was let down by the negative results, I was worried sick over my dad and the deteriorating phone calls I kept getting, and I was shocked at my husband's reaction to my *slightly* elevated wasp nest patrol. All in all, I was a complete and utter nutcase—full-on.

In the end, it worked out *eventually*. My dad recovered, thank God, but not without some repercussions of his own. Kevin and I patched ourselves up as well. Once we both cooled down and he got more details on what was going on with my father, he realized why I was stressed, and once I realized what was going on at his work (an unfounded fear that he might be losing his new job), I was also much more understanding. As we talked and I cried and we reconciled things, we thus dubbed that day forever as F.U.B.A.R. Friday and moved on. It was the most natural label for this epically horrible day and it stuck, so there you have it. At the very least, we learned how crucial it was to verbalize things before they became so huge.

On the fertility front, according to the nurse, I was to stop the progesterone and wait for my body to cycle on its own, and we would (as they say) lather, rinse, repeat that last cycle and try again. I was told that this could take as much a week or two, on August 1, 2008, I stopped the progesterone, bought a bottle of wine, and proceeded to try and drink myself to a happy place, relax a little, rest up, and wait.

Cut Short

Literally two days after all this chaos, my body cycled on its own, and two days after that, I began the drugs again. That was all the break I had… two stinking days. Two days to rest my body. Two days to try and get my hormones to settle down. Two measly days to enjoy my husband without the haze of injections and pills and tracking to cloud my mood. *Two freaking days.* I was still exhausted from the last cycle when we jump started the second one and I was much more emotionally raw. The protocol for this second cycle was pharmaceutically identical to the last cycle, but since I started out in a physical and mental deficit already, the side effects were noticeably worse. I began having migraines again, something that had not plagued me since my teenage years. I could not handle light of any kind, and my fatigue was incapacitating. I would sleep like the dead at night, even though I would wake-up sweating on most nights, and then spend the day walking around like a zombie as if I had never slept in my life. I had no energy, was bloated, my ovaries hurt, my head hurt, and overall, I felt like I had the flu (if the flu hit you at sixty miles an hour with a Mack truck, that is). By the time I got to my third day of injections, I sat there staring at the needle and started to cry. I was already so tired and so very weary, and I just simply could not do it. At that point, Kevin took it upon himself to actually give me

HEATHER D. NELSON

my injections to try and pitch in. He ordered pizza when I could not cook, he rubbed my feet to relax me, he covered up the windows with blankets to block out the light, and he officially gave up his favorite recliner for me to sleep in. In short, he did anything and everything within his power to make me feel better. I loved him *very much* for that. I had never seen him be so self-sacrificing before. I had never witnessed this ability of his to just serve me knowing full well that I could not reciprocate in anyway.

I went in to the doctor's office every other day for wand monitoring, and my ovaries behaved as they expected. We triggered and insemi-nated and things looked great. In fact, this cycle was described to me as being a classic and textbook cycle which should have been a good thing. But at the end of that cycle, again, we received a big fat negative on our beta. When I got that call, I was upstairs in my office and Kevin was downstairs in his. I was so despondent about the results and I did not know what to do. I asked the nurse if there was anything else I could do to help this process along and she suggested a few things I could try to manage the side effects and such, but in short, we were doing all we could and we just needed to keep on going. Geez. Keep on going. I suddenly couldn't breathe. That thought immediately made me feel as if a one hundred pound weight had been put in my hands. I was drained. My "break" in between was cut short and this cycle seemed to fly by and I had had no time to come to grips with the last month's failure, much less prepare for this month's failure. Even with all the positive thoughts and comments from the nursing staff, I was beat down and worn thin.

I hung up the phone from the doctor's office, I put my head down on my desk, and I began to cry. This was not a silent and graceful catharsis to relieve the stress of a month of drugs. Oh no, this was the loud, gut-wrenching, snot-inducing, dry heaving sobs of a woman who had hit the bitter end of her very frayed rope. I had now endured two months of major drugs back-to-back, a minor body surgery, a very sick father, and a total of ten months *solid* of some kind of medical poking, prod-ding, drug-sticking, bloodsucking, pharmacology-pushing treatment. I had not been to see my family in over a year or more, we had very little extra money to do much of anything other than pay for all the drugs, I was terrified to skip a month because "what if that was supposed to be our lucky month," but I was terrified of moving forward because I could not imagine how awful I would feel after another two months of this crap. I was horribly lonely too, and that all came to the surface as well. After being isolated from my family because of geography and isolated from our friends by circumstances and choice, I had never felt more alone and depressed in my life. Physically, I was beat up and worn down and had sort of let myself go. No haircuts, manicures, or even makeup on some days. Emotionally, I was completely spent, and it showed in every facet of my life. There were days I skipped showering altogether, I had no energy to do much of anything for myself and much less my husband. I was feeling completely and totally overwhelmed as all of the last year or more came to the surface. I was doing some *serious* crying. Moaning, gasping, wailing, heartbreaking, exhausting, unable to stand up kind of crying. I was so entrenched in my performance, in fact, that my husband heard me all the way downstairs in his office on the other end of the house. He silently came upstairs, pulled up a chair, and sat there holding my hand and rubbing my back while I sobbed and sobbed and sobbed some more. I felt as if I was crying the last of my strength out onto the floor in little puddles.

When I finally attempted to talk through the sobbing and nose blowing, I did equal parts confession and ranting. I ranted and raved at him about how lonely I was and how hard this was and how mad I was that it was not working. I told him that he could not understand what I was feeling because he did not have a uterus, and that it was not fair that I had to do all of this because of his jacked up swimmers. In truth, that was a completely unfair statement because he had lived every moment with me, but at that moment there was no stopping me, that dam had broken. I then started confessing my soul. I was the worst person ever for not being with my dad. I was scared to keep going and I was afraid we would spend all our money on this and have no money for adoption. I felt it was unfair for him to force this on me, because he could not handle adoption when it was not his body going through it. I continued that I was equally terrified to *stop* trying all this stuff, because what if that made our baby and we did not get the child we hoped for because I could not hack it. What would quitting say about me as a mother? Maybe that was why God had chosen to deny us all that time, because I was a major wuss-bag. The rant went on and on about how lonely I was and isolated I felt and how tired and physically beat up I was, and on and on and on I went. It was not a pretty sight. The whole thing lasted a good ten to fifteen minutes, and my volume and tears and anger increased incrementally as I went on.

Finally, out of sheer exhaustion, I slowed my pace enough for my husband to get in a word and he started begging and negotiating and promising all that was within his power to try and motivate me and lift me up. He agreed that we needed a break. He admitted that he finally saw, this past two months, how hard all this was on me physically and emotionally, and he would *not* ask me to do this indefinitely. He was more ready for adoption now and had a peace about it, and would be totally okay with that if that is what I wanted. However, he asked if I could give him two more cycles. After all, that would give us four cycles with Dr. Slater, who said we had really good odds in the three to six months after the surgery, and he did not want to totally throw those chances away if we could avoid it. After two more months if we still had no success, then no matter what, we would take off November and December to travel around over the holidays to see *all* my family. He even went on to sweeten the deal by saying that in January 2009, whether or not we decided to try again, or started adoption, would be entirely my choice and he would support us whatever way I wanted to go wholeheartedly. He even offered to pay for whatever extra supplementary support I needed to help get me through the next two cycles which, in my more cynical mind, I briefly considered that I "needed" weekly massages and pedicures, followed by new shoes and maybe some jewelry, but I rightly kept that to myself.

In the end, with all his verdant pleading, I did not have the heart to say no. Not then. Not yet. I could never really say no to my husband anyway, but that small voice in my head chimed in too. It said, "You know how hard adoption was for him, and the fact that he is recognizing that he is ready to start that process is huge. He needs to be sure, and you owe it to him to help give him that peace of mind too. After all, this is *both* your lives you're talking about, not your own. And honey, let's be real, you're much stronger than you realize and you'll be just fine." So I caved. I wiped my cheeks, blew my nose, hugged my husband, and somewhere inside myself found a small kernel of motivation to continue forward. At that moment, as I outwardly agreed to try two more cycles, I silently envisioned finding the owner of that small little voice in my head and smothering them with a pillow.

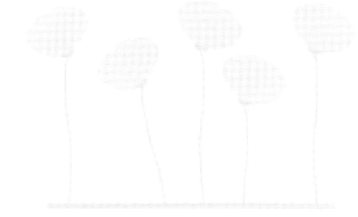

My Needle-Loving Guru

Apparently, my husband's offer to pay for whatever I needed to get me through the next two cycles was a serious offer. And by serious, I mean that the man *notoriously* known for his frugality in three states, actually opened up his wallet. He gladly, cheerfully even, paid for weekly visits to a fringe pseudo-medicinal Eastern practitioner of acupuncture, strictly on the recommendation of one person who said it *might* help with the side effects of my fertility shots. To the tune of sixty to seventy-five dollars per session no less, my husband footed the bill and encouraged me to attend as many times per week as I needed. This was a moment for quiet contemplation as I acknowledged how truly dedicated my penny-pinching husband was that he not only offered to pay, but as many times per week as I needed and, while I was out, stop by Starbucks and get my favorite drink too. My view of the world had truly turned on its side—my honey was shelling out superfluous money on a wing and a prayer, to try and help me maintain the bare minimum of sanity and emotional wherewithal that I had managed to hold on to thus far. I loved him a *lot* more for that, and perhaps felt slightly guilty that my emotional fragility had pushed him this far. I called and made my first appointment with the acupuncturist, all the while preparing to begin my new protocol of drugs and multiplue visits with my friend "Mr. Wand."

As the day approached for my first ever acupuncture appointment, I was not only totally apprehensive to go, but I was increasingly jittery because of the drugs. I mean, after all, if I really was looking for relaxation, why on earth would I sign up for *more* needles? I was already on the drugs for the third cycle with Dr. Slater, and the effects were definitely kicking in. I was sweating profusely, restless, had migraine headaches, constant fatigue, and general all over body aches and pains. I think I may have even been a little smelly too for that matter. On top of all that, I had a monstrous amount of baggage that I had been carrying around for the past six months and I was a virtual dam of irritation just ready to burst.

I arrived to a rather sterile, and corporate feeling, small waiting room that was slightly underwhelming. I was immediately handed a clipboard of paperwork to fill out on my "condition" and "areas of concern," which was very thorough. So thorough, in fact that I almost started to cry just filling it out. There was page after page of questions and check boxes about anything I may or may not have experienced in the entirety of my life. I was thinking to myself, "Geez, I'm a *mess*," especially since I had to check nearly every "symptom" listed as some area of my body that I had in the past, or was currently, struggling with. Literally from head (migraines) to toe (muscle cramps) there was hardly one single thing that I had not felt was a relevant symptom. It was embarrassing that my body felt so out of whack and even more so in that I never realized exactly how screwed up I was. When I completed the paperwork, I meekly handed it over and wished for that magical hole in the earth to open and swallow me. After that, the acupuncturist (Scott) took me back to a room that was very clean and sterile and "safe" looking, and we sat at a nice table and chatted for about half an hour. He described his own background, and how he had been involved with my fertility clinic for three years and had seen all manner of different women come through his office. In fact, the wonderful Dr. Slater would actually have Scott come into the clinic office and do treatments right on site for some IVF patients, which both surprised me and gave me some hope that perhaps this guy was not a total whack-job. He went on to ask gently probing questions about my fertility history and drug protocols. I did my best to answer him without giving him too much information. At times, however, TMI was exactly in order, and he was actually grateful for it. He said that the more detailed I could be, the more thoroughly and quickly he could treat my symptoms. After the Q&A session, it was time to hop up on the table and get started. That is when it got a little bizarre.

Bizarro

I had expected to strip down, don a sterile white sheet, and lay on my stomach while he put needles in my back. I also expected candles, soft music, and aromatherapy too. I guess I was expecting this to be like a massage or hot rock therapy or something. Instead, he instructed me to remain clothed, but kick off my shoes and socks and roll my pants up over my knees. That was a little relief since I wasn't sure I really *wanted* to get naked for yet another stranger. Once I was situated on the table, he began walking slowly around the table and taking my pulse in my wrist and ankles. Then, as if that wasn't odd enough, he asked me to stick out my tongue so he could see it. I was pretty sure this was a joke but he was serious.He continued circling the table but said nothing the whole time while quietly feeling my pulse on each wrist and ankle and feverishly taking notes. My patience was growing a bit thin with the anticipation. What the heck was he writing down anyway!?!

He then popped his head up from his clipboard and asked me, flat out, if I had been feeling as if the world had turned the gravity on super-high in the mornings. As odd of a question as it was, it perfectly described how I had been feeling with all the injections and stress. He went on to ask me if I had been feeling hot more often or if my heart felt as if it had skipped a beat and then would rush to catch up. He even asked if I ever had dizzy spells. I was able to quickly remember that those exact things had happened at least once or twice per cycle of meds and the dizzy spells and hot flashes, in particular, had been more and more frequent. I was weirded out beyond measure that this *guy* was able to pinpoint and describe my feelings better than I was. I was more weirded out that he did all that after feeling the pulse in my ankle and observing the color and texture of my tongue. The whole thing was odd.

Luckily, needle guru Scott explained why he was doing what he was doing, and how it worked. In short, he explained that in Chinese medicine they teach that all emotional responses were actually triggered by some area within the body that was off-kilter somehow. Anxiety and stress were heart related, anger and rage another area, and so on and so forth. In my case, he went on to enlighten, my body was working over-time on the inside with all the hormones I was on. I was effete because of this extra work, and all the overabundance of energy my body was using to process the hormones had nowhere to go except into the form of heat. The excess heat further altered my energy levels, and then all of that was stimulating the emotional response of anxiety and stress and that general overwhelmed feeling. In other words, it was a vicious cycle that I was stuck in. Believe it or not, this guy had (in under twenty-five minutes) pinpointed and perfectly described my exact feelings for the previous six-plus months, and had gone on further to not only justify my emotional anxiety and reactions, but excuse them. He even compli-mented me for the fact that I had gone for so long and handled things as well as I had without cracking up. I was too ashamed to tell him that I had not, in fact, handled it that well and that my appointment with him was a testament to just how desperate my poor husband was to find relief. I was dumbfounded that this guy really knew what he was talk-ing about. And yet, *with all that*, I was still skeptical, but by now, I was headlong into the process and it was time for (insert dramatic music here)* *the needles.*

I was already on the table with my pants rolled over my knees, but Scott added that I needed to roll my shirt up under my bra, thus expos-ing my rib cage. He started with my right hand, then right leg/foot, then left leg/foot, hand, ribs, and face, placing needles methodically throughout each location. All told, he only put a few needles in me and I did not feel them go in at all. The fact that there was no real pain involved was some relief. I am a big sissy wuss-bag about physical pain. As he continued circling around me putting needles in, my whole body started to get tense and I began to feel increasingly anxious.Suddenly I

HEATHER D. NELSON

was freezing cold, which was weird because I was literally sweating hot when I arrived at his office. I did not say anything to Scott because I was afraid he would think I was weird. I decided to let him keep working and I silently hoped that he would not notice my tension. By the time he was done, I was on the verge of tears for no reason at all, save that I was a ball of strained anxiety. So much so that I feel confident I was practically levitating off the table with the sheer force of my stress level. I did not want to breakdown like some emotional wreck on his table. I did my best to maintain my outward composure and I held my breath and silently begged him to leave the room before the dam broke. He finished placing all the needles and told me that he was going to leave me alone to rest in this position for about twenty minutes.He said that he would be back to check on me, but that if I needed him to just call out for him. He set the hippie tree-hugger music CD to a low volume and turned down the lights before leaving. I was still holding my breath, waiting for him to get out before the floodgates opened. Finally, he headed for the door and before stepping out, he turned and intuitively said, "Oh by the way, there are a lot of tears shed in this room. Do not be ashamed or afraid of them. Crying is a really good sign and I want you to feel free to feel whatever you feel. *This* is my job." At that point, the floodgates opened wide. Scott walked out, closed the door, and I proceed to cry for a solid ten minutes.

It was not that loud, hard crying that you do quickly and then it is over, but rather it was a slow, steady stream of tears as I laid there on the table. The tears just flowed down my cheeks and pooled into my ears and onto the table as if a faucet had been turned on. It was the most relaxing cry I had ever had. My body was shaking all over and I was praying to God over and over. I prayed, or rather begged, God to help me. "Please take this burden away from me…please help me to *not* be so overwhelmed all the time…give me strength to push forward through these next two rounds for my husband…give me grace…give me peace…give me understanding…" and on and on I went. Just silently crying, shaking, and praying. It was cathartic to say the least, and I felt a little embarrassed that it took seventy-five dollars, two hours of needles, and twinkly hippie music to accomplish this. Finally, after about ten minutes of solid crying and praying and shaking, my tears finally stopped. At almost the same moment, my body started getting goose bumps all over, and small electrical-like feelings around the areas of each of the needles. It was not painful at all and in fact, was incredibly relaxing and I was finally able to stop shaking as I sat there and studied what I was feeling. Then, the palms of my hands, which were face down on the table next to me, began to feel warm. Not that sweating, internal hot feeling, but more of an external sensation. It was as if there was sunlight streaming through a window and warming my palms that way… as if they were radiating heat and glowing somehow. Suddenly, I did not feel cold at all, or hot for that matter. I was thinking to myself how I must be crazy and that there was no way I could possibly have felt all that in such a short amount of time. Before I could even process all the sensations, Scott came back in the room and asked how I was doing. I mentioned the hot palms feeling, and he said that was a good sign that my body was releasing some of that pent-up heat. He said he wanted to tweak all the needles a little bit to see if he could offer me more relief, and I agreed. At that point, he walked all around my body again, adjusting the needles. As he circled me, I was lying there relaxing until he reached my right foot. I had one needle sticking in the middle of the top of my foot. He did something with that needle, and my foot suddenly spasmed and my *entire right leg* jumped up and I felt this electrical pulse run all the way up the right side of my body to my jaw, which loudly popped! Just as I was yelling, "What the heck was that?", he yelled, "Bingo, Yahtzee, there it is, finally!" I looked at him like he was a crazy person and said, "Finally What?" He told me that this reaction was my body finally releasing a huge burst of that trapped energy inside me. It was, apparently, the reaction he was looking for and he was glad to see it. I was freaked totally out. He even said that not many people had such a severe reaction, and that I must have been feeling like a ticking time bomb for months now. I laughed a little because I *was* a walking time bomb of emotions. The weirdness factor of this whole appointment had reached a whole new level by now. Not only did this guy *nail* my feelings to the letter, but my body had done everything he wanted it to do, and then this weird spasm thing with my leg happened.

It did not hurt, but did scare the crap out of me. Once he completed adjusting the needles, and reveling in his own success with my funky leg thing, he left me once again to relax. As he stepped out and closed the door, I suddenly had an overwhelming urge to go potty. Or rather, I had to pee like a racehorse! I was supposed to lay there another five minutes with the needles and *relax*, and the whole time I was afraid I would wet my pants. This time, instead of praying for God to give me strength, I began to pray to God for bladder control! When Scott finally returned and removed the needles I was dying. I felt like it took him an eternity to work his way around me and I began to contemplate how bad it would *really* hurt if I ran to the bathroom with a few needles still left in me. Finally he finished up and without any prompting from me, he said, "The bathroom is through that door." This guy was freakishly in tune with me. I briefly considered asking him how he knew I had to go badly, but was already halfway down the hall and unbuttoning my pants in the process. Thus ended my very first acupuncture appointment.

Scott explained that I had reacted much as he expected. He said I would definitely see some changes in my body and emotions over the coming days, and that he wanted to see me the following week. I tried to pry out of him any details on what I could expect, but he would not divulge *what* changes I would see. He guaranteed me that things should be different now. He laughed a little and said I was, indeed, wound up tighter than a spring and he would focus on releasing all that tension in our next few sessions. He also told me that the urge to use the bathroom was a common reaction to my body releasing all the toxins as my muscles relaxed. That was just a gross thought to contemplate.

As I left his office, two hours later and seventy-five dollars lighter, I did notice a few things. I was not hot. I walked into his appointment near sweating hot, but now was comfortable. I also was not feeling as emotionally fragile. I was still tired, but did not feel quite so overwhelmed by life. I did not know if I accounted all of that to my right foot doing the involuntary cha-cha on the table or the emotional reaction to the whole ordeal. At the very least, I was glad I went and I was intrigued enough to make a follow-up appointment and go back in a week as instructed.

Finally, that night, I contentedly slept and actually woke up feeling more rested and more human than I had in months.

Bizarro: the Sequel

My following appointment a week later was not near as eventful, but still had its quirks. I drove there thinking I was much more mentally prepared the second time around. After all, by now I knew what to expect and I was almost cocky in thinking this would be a cakewalk. Boy howdy, was I wrong.

I showed up and, again, my needle-loving guru asked me questions about how I had felt over the last week. I was honest in that I had only felt one hot flash, which was a mild one. I also told him that I had slept better in the last week than I had all month and I had not had a single migraine during the entire drug protocol thus far. These were all huge accomplishments and I mentally gave myself a gold star for being such a good sport about all this bizarro Chinese medicine. Scott concurred that my responses were exactly what he was hoping to see. He did not want to plant anything in my head which is why he would not voice those hopes to me last week. He was glad to hear that I had responded so well and returned for more. Then it was time to begin again so I rolled up my pants, hiked up my shirt, and hopped up on the table.

He started out, like before, checking my pulse. Or rather, as he explained it in more detail this time, checking the "spaces in between my pulse" and checking my "fertility pulse." Now, I was not aware that my body had more than one pulse to begin with, but he was the freaky Eastern medicine expert, so I just shut my pie hole and waited for his official word. He was slightly relieved by what he was feeling in my wrist and ankles. Apparently my fertility pulse was much stronger this time than it was a week ago. He told me that he intentionally did *not* tell me a week ago that it was very weak because he did not want to worry me. I guess he knew me fairly well, because I would have utterly panicked over the concept of a *weak fertility pulse*. Fertility pulse, however, was greatly increased in the last week, and he was glad and we moved on. Scott also noticed that my energy level was stronger and in general, there was huge improvement in my condition. But even with all that positive feedback, he still noticed an underlying current of tension in my body. When he told me this, I looked at him, cocked up one eyebrow and said, "Well, duh!" He laughed and said that he realized that I was taking daily injections equivalent to a hormonal pregnant teenager, and that it might cause a *wee bit of stress* in the process. But he felt that the cause of my tension was deeper and actually hindering some of his efforts. He then cocked his head and commented on my giant Starbucks cup sitting next to my shoes on the floor. I followed his gaze over just as he said "Maybe next time, we save the gallon of caffeine for *after* the treatment?"

Now, as a side bar, I am a normal, red-blooded American woman and as such, I love me some Starbucks! Their coffee is the bomb, the macchiatos are heaven in a cup, and on a day when I am hot and on the go, their black iced tea is the perfect oasis in life to keep me going. As I was already undertaking acupuncture to try and find the jelly-filled zen center in my life and be more calm, I felt that this required merry bushels of caffeine to aid in my relaxation. Alas, my needle dude asked that I leave the bucket-o-caffeine until *after* my acupuncture and I agreed, but not without asking why. He noticed the tension in my pulse and felt it might be *slightly* askew because of the caffeine. I agreed, again, and he began the needle portion of the show. For the most part, all needles were the same, one in each hand, one in each foot, several around my ankles and lower legs, and then one in between my eyes, "just for fun" he said. I chuckled and thought to myself, "*Cause needles in between my eyes are fun!?!*"

During my last appointment, the first part of this show was pretty low-key, but when he came in to tweak the pins, my right foot did an involuntary cha-cha off the table and freaked me out. He promised it would not be that way this time around and yet, from the moment he put that needle in my right foot, it felt like it was on the verge of spazzing out again. I hoped it would calm down in time. Again, Scott set me up like a pin-cushioned Jello mold and I proceeded to sit very still while he put on the funky mood-music and let me chill for twenty minutes. As he left the room, I took a moment to take some personal stock in my situation. I was not crying this time at all, and I did not even feel the need. It only took five minutes for my body to relax this time instead of ten or fifteen. I was not having the hot/cold flashes like last time, but was above all, my right foot and leg were *pissed off.*

During the first fifteen minutes, my foot felt like it was on the verge of a massive charley horse. I did not dare "stretch it out" because I was skewered with tiny needles that would surely puncture something vital should I have moved at all. After a few minutes of this, my right leg, *again,* started making involuntary movements; little jerks and spasms, all on its own, despite all my efforts to remain still. I was seriously trying to remember where he had put all the needles, and wondering if my little spasms would somehow shove a needle even deeper. Finally, toward the end, my foot finally released, and my leg got quiet and I was able to relax. Enter the guru.

It was then time for the "tweaking" portion of the show, and he started with my ribs and worked his way down. The needle in my hands hurt like a mother which he commented on as being one of the most tightly wound areas in me that day. I sarcastically thought, *gee thanks for that note to the obvious... cause my HANDS are why I'm here.* The rest of the needle adjustments were fine, but when he got to my feet I simply told him, "My foot has only just stopped doing the cha-cha from your last go-round with it, and I really do not want a repeat of last weeks weirdness. What say we ignore that needle for the second round." He laughed and agreed, and tweaked the rest of my needles and let me chill for another five minutes before returning to de-pin me.

We chatted afterward and discussed when my next appointment should be. He said that some women he wanted to see *on* the day of their insemination, because he needed to "help their fertility" a little and offer more support in that area. But for me, while it could not hurt, he was not sure it was necessary at all. My fertility pulse had increased greatly and was pretty strong this time. I gave myself a mental gold star. However, he felt my bigger stumbling block was all the caged up tension. Scott felt that keeping me "unwound" after the insemination would benefit me more than anything else. I couldn't help but laugh at the idea that *I* of all people might be *a little wound up.* We discussed my right foot/leg, and he said there is an acupuncture "tack" they can put in there that remains all day and all night to help, but he felt that was too much too soon. The idea of walking around looking like I fell into a tackle box was wholly unappealing, so I agreed with him *vehemently* on this point. In fact, I further commented that I was glad my right foot did not have such a dramatic moment this time, and he said, "Yes, and in general, you will notice that when we get you finally leveled out, you will be a little less dramatic overall."

Me? *Dramatic?* Surely you jest!

In the end, it was a good appointment. I slept really well that night again, and made an appointment for the following Tuesday, agreeing to forego my five dollars of "heaven in a cup" until *after* the zen master was done checking my multiple pulses. The best part of this appointment though was when he actually suggested that the *best* thing we could do to improve our chances at the time of insemination was to have my husband rub my feet the entire twenty minutes that I had to lay there post-IUI and wait for all the swimmers to "hit bottom." He said it would help relax me and that the points in the foot/ankle would stimulate blood flow to the uterine area that would be beneficial. I conveyed this suggestion to my husband and he said, without one iota of hesitation, "Okay!"

Now *that alone* was worth sixty-five bucks. *Prescribed foot rubs!*

I had my third acupuncture session after my insemination. He said I was responding really well, and even I could fully attest to how much easier this cycle was as far as the side effects were concerned. He put the needles in different locations to "lift and support" a pregnancy should I have one, but then told me that I did not need to come back until our next cycle started, *if* it started, that is. I walked out of there feeling quite proud of myself with multiple mental "gold stars" for responding well and being a good sport overall. *Go me,* I thought.

Two Weeks All Over Again

I spent the next week staying really busy with decorating my church for fall and wrapping up my work duties, since I was officially, and gleefully, joining the ranks of stay-at-home wives. I was impressed at how well I was doing at not freaking out over my two-week waiting period this time and I thought to myself, *that is another gold star on my mental chart.* Go me. I was nervous but also thoroughly excited about the prospect of no longer working. I was a little anxious about all the perceived free time on my hands, but more than anything, I was looking forward to being a *wife* and taking care of my house and husband for a change. It was another one of those "kinda weird timing things" though. Kevin and I had jointly made the decision for me to quit about one and a half weeks prior to this. Then, the day *after* our decision, we watched the movie "Facing the Giants." In this movie, a man tells a story of two farmers who were both in desperate need for rain. They both prayed fervently to God to send rain, but only one prepared his fields to receive it, thus showing a greater faith. It was a little prophetic for me. Here I sat, quitting my job for no good reason other than I wanted to and I felt it was time, and yet I was not pregnant and we had no kids, save our two crazy fur-babies. I liked to think that I was preparing my fields for rain.

Over the previous four-plus years, we had changed our lifestyle dramatically. I went from punching an office job clock, to working from home, to stay-at-home wife. Financially, we went from living on credit cards, to being almost totally debt-free and living on a cash basis with plans for savings and retirement. Even my husband had gone from being sorely underpaid, to obtaining a few raises, and then even making the jump to self-employed and earning much closer to what he was worth. In general, we had been slowly adjusting our lifestyles to prepare for a family all this time, and now I was taking that final step in quitting my job. I was seriously hoping it was portentous, too, that we would get our baby soon, but I said to myself, either way, I *will* love God. If this cycle got us a baby or not, or if we had to adopt or not, God was King in our lives and the results of this would not change that. Either way, my fields were prepared I had planned all I could and I was ready for my baby now. Clearly, God had other plans.

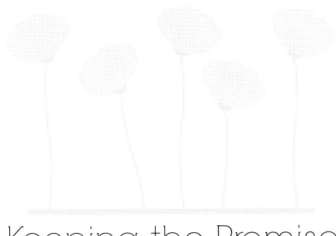

Keeping the Promise

On October 6, I got the call I had been dreading—a confirmed negative pregnancy test. I had already begun to feel my menstrual cycle coming on, so I was expecting the bad news. Nonetheless it was discouraging. During that call, Missy (the very sweet nurse) was sympathetic that we had yet again failed a cycle and said it was time to consult with the doctor to determine the next course of action. Apparently having three "classic" and "textbook" cycles with good response, multiple eggs, good sperm count, and still failing to conceive is cause to regroup and get a new game plan. I was instantly, and to my very core, terrified. Terrified that the doctor would tell us there is nothing more she can do and we are on our own; terrified that she would tell us IVF is our only hope, which we could not afford and had even less odds; terrified that we had to face the inevitable end of our road, mourn the loss of our biological child, and face adoption which, as it happens, I was not as ready as I thought. I was terrified. Terrified that the doctor would tell us there was still hope, that we need to keep trying; terrified that she'd require more tests, more painful surgeries, but give us hope we would never get off this crazy roller coaster. I was terrified that we would decide to keep trying and go through a repeat of the last year's hope and failure and heartbreak a few more times. I was terrified.

- Terrified to keep trying because of the pain, heartbreak, financial strain, waiting, and time lost.
- Terrified to quit trying because what if the *next one* is the one that gets us our baby.
- Terrified to do nothing and start the adoption process, only to have our hearts broken again.
- Terrified to do anything.
- Terrified to do nothing.

I did not want to meet with the doctor. I wanted to crawl in that magical body-swallowing hole in the earth and disappear. That hole was simply never around when I needed it! Then, perfectly timed as always, that still small voice in my head that I had learned to both love and hate told me that this meeting with the doctor was the right thing to do. I did not even bother to argue with "the voice" this time. I scheduled the meeting for the next day (the 7th), and immediately scheduled a meeting with Pastor Jeff for the 8th as well. I knew this was going to be a *big* decision-making period for us and I wanted to feel as prepared as possible. The next day, off we went to the doctor's consult. Admittedly, it was more out of obligation, because my little head voice buddy was telling me it was the right thing to do. I felt it better to arm ourselves with as much information as possible to make an educated choice, but still I did not *want* to go. I was thinking to myself the whole way to the doctor's office, "I'll ask the good questions, dutifully take notes, and intelligently discuss our choices. I will even try to find my stiff upper lip somewhere and bring it along with me so the doctor does not see me break down into an utter blob of snot and tears." But in my heart, I was terrified and did not want to be there. I was brave on the outside, but had inwardly melted into a puddle of gutless wonder.

When Kevin and I arrived at Dr. Slater's office, hand in hand, I felt like I knew what to expect. I suspected she would come in, all business-like, and review our history of total failure from our big fat file. Then she'd lay out the options for us, very clinically, and look down her nose at us for wasting so much of her time on useless IUI's. Finally, I expected, she would sit back in her giant chair and cross her arms behind that enormous desk and wait for us to decide to do IVF like we should have done from the beginning. I was pleasantly surprised, though. Dr. Slater was surprisingly the opposite of my expectations. She was not all business-like, and instead she was *very* compassionate and mild-mannered in her approach. This spelled disaster for my stiff upper lip.

First, she reviewed our history of each of our three cycles. She did not review them like a postmortem of disappointing efforts though; she looked at where they succeeded. She focused on the good sperm counts, the great egg response, etc. It was refreshing, the way she made all our botched baby-making somehow seem positive. Then she laid out all our options as she saw them. She confirmed that we had shown great response to the injectibles and thus had good cycles really. She went on to state that there was no *known* reason for us to not *eventually* succeed. *Eventually*. She said that we technically could do some exploratory surgery to look for endometriosis or some other as yet unfound cause to all this. My heart skipped a beat at the idea of more surgery. Dr. Slater quickly followed her statement up by telling us that she saw no reason for surgery, as I had no history or symptoms, and otherwise seemed healthy. She did not think we needed any extra surgeries or "tests" at all in fact, which she made a point to state. She did agree to recheck my thyroid levels for me, but I felt that was more to put me at ease because I asked for it. All in all, she left the choice of where to go firmly in our very yellow-bellied and incapable hands. We could either:

- Continue doing what we're doing, but be more aggressive with the drugs to slightly increase our chances of having more mature follicles and higher risk of multiple birth.

- Switch to IVF, and then she broke down the cost, options, financing, etc.

- Dial back our efforts to Clomid and timed "fun" for a few months to take a breather and give me a physical and emotional break.

- Quit altogether for the next three months and then restart after the first of the year.

- Quit altogether… period.

She fully supported us for whatever we wanted to do, and I was glad she did not push any one option over another. At this point, I asked all kinds of questions, and she addressed each one fully and with both expertise and compassion. After dodging around a bit, I finally asked the big question that had been plaguing me for over a year. And yes, I did breakdown a little when I asked her "Why?" How had we gotten pregnant with our Peanut with the lowest dosage of Clomid and timed "baby dancing," but now could not hit pay dirt with all we'd done in the past year or more? With all the surgeries and injections and IUIs and more, *why* was it not happening for us? As I wiped the tears off my cheek and Kevin squeezed my hand, I held my breath, waiting to hear her response. She was very gentle in her answer and was understanding of my emotional response. She said that there was no known reason why things had not worked in all this time other than, "Sometimes, these unexplainable things simply just happen." She went on to encourage us further that we had been having good responses to all the treatments thus far and it still *could* happen with more perseverance, but that, in short, it was decision-making time. Inwardly, I cringed at the thought of needing "more perseverance." I did not think I had any more perseverance in me. I was tired and hurt and strung out to the point of not being able to do anymore. At that point, my husband and I had a very brief, but oddly succinct, interchange between us. He, who had previously begged me for two more cycles, was suddenly perfectly willing to stop altogether at this point after realizing how taxed I was physically and emotionally. He was completely ready for adoption if that was my choice and he would support my decision in whatever I decided. In other words, with the doctor's kind support and my husband's gentle understanding, I was in the hot seat to make this choice on my own. I thought to myself, *Gee thanks, you big bunch of cowards!*

I had spent a considerable amount of time in thought about this very moment and had already prayed to God a lot for guidance. I had not received much feedback from the Man Upstairs and as the good doctor and my husband both stared silently at me, I felt no closer to making a decision than I was before. However, in the back of my mind, I suddenly heard that still small voice, "You made a promise. You promised your husband two more cycles and you still owe him one." Man, did I hate that voice in my head at that moment. I mean, here was my chance to bail out of this maze of emotional torture once and for all with no judgment against me, and *now* the stupid voice chooses to pop-up and throw its two cents in. *Now!?* Talk about impeccable timing. Alas, I could not argue with *the voice*. I *had* promised. My husband was and is a man of great integrity, and integrity is of great importance to him. And in truth, this journey was not my burden to bear alone, but a journey paired with my marriage to a man who loved me unendingly and without fail at every turn. Surely, I owed it to him to give him that one last promised cycle that he had begged me for so fervently. Surely I could find it in myself to just muddle through one more month… for him. And *that* was exactly what I decided. One more to fulfill the promise, ease my conscience, assuage my guilt, whatever you want to call it, but that small voice in my head gave me a verbal high-five as I announced to my husband and the doctor, "Okay, we'll do one more cycle." I added a small caveat to my decision though. I said, "Let's blow the roof off this thing and be super aggressive and then call it quits for a few months." To my surprise, everyone agreed.

We agreed that this last protocol would be more aggressive pharmaceutically to try and increase the number of follicles we had, and give ourselves the best possible chances. We added a male fertility supplement to the mix for my husband as well, to up the odds some micro amount. I would continue, if not increase, my acupuncture appointments to manage the side effects. My drugs, this last time, consisted of higher Clomid and higher doses of injectables, with more frequent ultrasounds to monitor my progress. Then we would trigger to ovulate and do an IUI as previously was done. Since we were going very aggressively with it, Dr. Slater agreed that instead of aiming for only two mature follicles this time, we would shoot for four or more. We even had to sign off that we acknowledged our risk of triplets, but it was a risk I was glad to take and one that the doctor supported, given our history.

My husband felt good about my decision, although fearful of me giving birth to a baseball team. I felt a sense of peace in knowing that we would have then tried *everything* we could feasibly afford before throwing in the proverbial towel, and that I had also fulfilled my promise to Kevin as well. My decision went a little beyond just this round of drugs though. I had decided, that after this last cycle, we would stop for the holidays. I needed the break and wanted to know that I could enjoy the holidays with my family without this stress and chaos on me. I told my husband that when the New Year came along, pending I didn't change my mind, we would do Clomid and timed intercourse only, and move full-bore toward adoption at the same time. Kevin agreed fully…just as he had promised he would. Dr. Slater even went ahead and gave me the Clomid scrip we would need for the future months, "just in case." At the time, it sort of felt like planning for failure, but at the same time, I felt armed and more ready to move on. I had walked into that appointment in knots worrying about any and every possibility. I walked out of there feeling confident in our decision and at least at peace with the choice I had made.

The next day we met with Pastor Jeff again, and the confirmation of our decision was immediately made apparent to us. We sat down and he asked us where we were in our journey. We told him that we had met with Dr. Slater and after all our discussions, had decided to do one more cycle, full-bore, and then quit for a time, if not quit altogether. Pastor Jeff nearly jumped out of his chair with excitement at that. He said he had already prayed for us and felt strongly that we should quit and was going to counsel us to do just that. The fact that we already felt that way and had made that call on our own was even more confirmation all-around that it was the right choice to make. He acknowledged that he knew we wanted a baby very badly, but that all the medical treatments, drugs, tests, money, surgeries, and more were taking a serious toll on our everyday lives. We had both started to retreat from life a bit, me out of defense and Kevin out of necessity and support. Pastor Jeff felt that anything we did that pulled us away from serving God and living our lives this much was not a healthy thing, and he was glad we had made our choice. We talked more about adoption and our mixed feelings about it, and then Pastor Jeff addressed my need to keep the promise to my husband and acknowledged that it was a good intention as a wife to want to respect my husband's wishes. As it stood, we all felt it was a good choice to move forward with one more cycle and then take a break. In other words, we all agreed this was the time to *go big or go home,* and with that, I decided it was time for an e-mail to our families:

Hey guys,

Kevin and I have spent quite some time the past few weeks discussing our path to parenthood and what our plans are for the future. In the process, we met with our specialist and have consulted with our pastor as well. After a lot of thought, tears, and prayer, we agreed that our road is coming to an end. We are attempting one last cycle with the specialist and drugs and such. With our doctor's blessing, we are getting very aggressive with this cycle to give us the best possible odds. We are also beginning the early education process on adoption. If this cycle fails, we will move headlong forward into the adoption process and just let nature take its course.

This is certainly not an easy decision for us to make. We factored in a lot of things like finances, emotional/physical strain, timing, and more. We've been trying, in total, for nearly two years; one whole year after the miscarriage. Even though I had unknown scar tissue, I have been on some kind of treatment/ hormone/procedure/etc. for a year solid with twelve consecutive months of negative results. I'm drained. Financially, we've managed to do all this on a nearly one hundred percent cash basis, but each cycle has cost us three thousand dollars or more, and IVF would be fifteen thousand dollars. With our savings drained, we would have to go into debt to continue doing what we're doing and when push comes to shove, we both agreed we did not want to go into debt for this, and would rather save our money for the adoption road than spend another year on what we're doing with no guarantees. All of those issues and more have been poured into our decision.

We will need a lot of prayer this month. With the cycle being very aggressive for our "go all out" effort, it will be physically more demanding on me. Please pray that we get through this gracefully with as little pain as possible. Beyond that, if this last ditch attempt fails, please pray that God heals our hearts from what will be a huge loss. While we still have the possibility for a biological child of our own, the odds are not in our favor. We hope that if this is what our path should be, God will make the adoption process as easy/fast/painless as possible for us, and help us accept that road to parenthood with as much desire and hope as we did this one.

I've already started the meds for this last round. We'll likely do the IUI on or around the 20th and will know for sure if it succeeded or failed on or around the November 3. We are crossing our fingers that our holiday travels come with a few extra "passengers!" I know that you all have been thinking of us and we appreciate it greatly. If you could manage a few more prayers this month on our behalf, it would mean the world.

Somehow, that e-mail to our family and friends made everything more "real" and very, very finite. Tears streamed down my face as I typed it and it took me a good hour to finally hit "send" on that message. I admitted to Kevin that I felt like a quitter somehow. I finally understood how some women would try and fight for five or ten years for this. I had learned how each month there is such hope that you will win the battle, but that I could not do it anymore and I really felt it was time to give up. I still felt good about our choice, but I felt equal amounts of shame and sorrow at my own weakness. I was proud of myself as a wife for respecting my husband's needs in this, and proud of our marriage and how we had maintained our relationship so well through all these many months/years of treatments, but I felt a sense of failure for not making it "work" yet. But one thing was very clear. No matter what, we would love God and trust Him. Failed cycle––love God. Adoption avenue—love God. Our hearts would break, but we would *know* God would get us through it, since He'd already pulled us through this much. We were definitely throwing one more Hail Mary pass with infertility treatments, but we did so knowing full well that God was our receiver in the end zone and if it were meant to happen, He would make it so… not us.

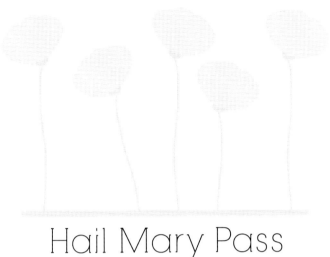

Hail Mary Pass

This last cycle was different from all previous ones in almost every possible way. The drugs themselves were much the same protocol as previous months, with the exception of higher dosages. The process itself was still the same. Take the drugs on appropriate days, do injections, visit the doctor every other day for probing ultrasounds and monitoring etc., etc., etc., ad nauseam, and then trigger, inseminate, and wait.

But for all the familiarity of this cycle, there was much that I was not prepared for. I was no longer working, so I felt confident I could manage the side effects better. But just as my cycle was beginning, all sorts of weird things cropped up that utterly *packed* my schedule which made the side effects of the drugs horrendous. I scheduled an acupuncture session that had me feeling like I was a rotisserie chicken but even with that I was sapped of all energy. The cycle turned out to be no easier than any of the others. If anything, it was much more emotional for me owing to the knowledge that this was our *last* opportunity. I tried my best to rest and not overtax my body and still, the migraines were awful, my fatigue was at record levels, and my emotions and mental state were fantastically fragile. I would vacillate between exhausted and weepy with a hair-trigger temper, to snippy and angry because of the headaches. At the heart of it though, all of that was a symptom of the fact that my body was *ready* to be done with all this mess, and my spirit was equally finished, even if my heart wasn't willing to admit it. I was in a personal state of conflict over the decision I had so confidently made just weeks beforehand. I tried to take things in stride as much as I could, and my sainted husband did his level best to cater to me as much as he was able. Secretly, I think he was holding his breath though, as was I.

We had decided this would be our final cycle and that decision had not waivered. We would go aggressive with the meds, aim for mega-number of follicles, and basically blow out all the stops. But at the end of the day, this was to be our reproductive swan song—our Hail Mary pass. And yet, with all our prayer, discussion, consults, and big plans, I felt no more prepared to end our journey than before. I had it in my head that I would be *relieved* to have decided to stop all the drugs and surgeries and treatments, but I was not. I felt as if *admitting* defeat was somehow *accepting* defeat, and thus *inviting* defeat. In the back of my mind, I began to question my confidence in our decision. Had I really heard that small voice telling me to do this one more time… or was I deluding myself into believing this was the right thing for my own selfish reasons?

Frustration and Doubt

At our final sonogram to monitor the progress of this cycle, we both went into the appointment with high expectations and equally high fears. Up until now, my cycle had been, again, textbook. Good lining, good follicle response, etc. All things pointed toward a record successful insemination, which I had unknowingly and desperately held on to as my reason for putting myself through it all. After all, what was a few weeks of torturous drugs if it meant a half-dozen good follicles, optimum chances at conception, and a fully clear conscience when it was all said and done? My husband, on the other hand, walked into that appointment utterly panic-stricken that we would have four or more huge follicles, end up inseminating and implanting all of them, and be the next couple on the local news for having a small litter of children in one single birthing, thus instantly going from a couple of D.I.N.K.s to married, one income, and six kids!

When I hopped up on to the table and they began to sonogram me to determine my follicle count, we were both wrong. Way wrong. I only had three follicles that's it: three. The same number, or even less, than previous lower dosage cycles, and no chance to have more by waiting longer. Three sad little insignificant follicles had taken the clear lead and grown to mammoth proportions and were ready to burst. My husband almost danced a jig with relief which would have been a funny visual at any other time. I, on the other hand, was utterly, completely, without reservation, pissed off! I think I even said to the sonographer, "*Are you freaking kidding me?* Only three? I feel like a bloated piece of crap and there is only **three**? " She snickered and said, "Yep, just three, although we do see a good amount of fluid, which would explain your bloated feeling. You likely are *mildly* overstimulated." That did *not* make me feel better at all. I mean, sure we had decided this was our final big push to try and conceive, and yes, we both felt it was time to stop, and *yes already,* I was the one mainly pushing the "I cannot take it anymore" angle on things. But for cryin' out loud, *three!?!?!?!?*

We scheduled our trigger and insemination appointments, checked out, and headed back home. I was steaming out of my ears from frustration. I felt totally gypped somehow and in truth, I had really gypped myself. I had it in my head, all bundled up nice and neat, that we would make this one big huge effort, have massive follicle response and optimum chances, and then if we failed, I would be mentally prepared to let go and move onto adoption knowing I had given it my all. It was so nice and neat I could have put a freaking bow around it. But now I was thinking, *"Well, what if I did* not *give it my all? What if I can do more drugs next time to really up the follicle count? What if one more month is what we need?"* In short, I was doubting my decision. Of course I expressed some of this undersurface seething to my mister, and he was quick to not only reinforce the *why* of our decision to stop, but to point out that—in truth—I would have these doubts no matter what. He said, "Think about it, is there really *any* number of follicles that would make you happy with our ending this road?" Of course the answer was a resounding no. And that still small voice in my head told me he was right. I really, *really* hated that voice!

I conceded though that my husband was right and there was nothing more for me to do at this point but push on. We triggered that night and went in as scheduled for our final insemination, which was relatively uneventful and frankly "old hat" at that point. Other than being *really* painful due to the extra fluid that was now keeping me from getting comfortably into my favorite pair of jeans, there was not much to write home about. After that, it was close to Halloween and time to wait out the next two weeks and plan to move forward. Our final two weeks… the last fourteen days of insanity we would ever have again as far as we knew. I could hear the swans a-singing in the background. Elvis was leaving the building and the fat lady was serenading him out the door. This was it.

Final Wait

I had big plans for those fourteen days to keep myself mega-busy. I was a little proud of myself in fact, for the way I was handling things and I added a mental gold star to my chart of self-appreciation. I volunteered to help at our church's Halloween bonfire, I invited a couple over for dinner one night, heck, I even planned on surprising my husband by remodeling his entire office while he was out of town on a business trip. I was serious that I was going to be pro-active, stay busy, and attack this final two-week wait with all the ferocity I could muster. That way, I reasoned, I could still feel as if I had done all I could do and be able to just finally let it all go. Surely that crazy train of illogical thinking makes perfect sense. Pack my schedule with social events so I can feel superfertile. Yep, no crazy there!

The Halloween gig was awful. It was a bonfire at night and it was freezing cold outside. I have no tolerance for the cold on a *good* day, but much less when I am already so run down. I was horridly bloated from all the drugs and meds, and still very physically taxed out. When I was not running around trying to be helpful, I spent a good part of that night about doubled-over in a chair from cramping and bloating and pressure. I was so tired I could barely *stand* by the time it was all over and apparently a few friends noticed and ratted me out to my husband. When Kevin discovered how much pain I was in, he literally led me to the car and took me home. I think he was pissed at me for pushing myself, but if he was, he did not say it.

The dinner was the emotional equivalent of a sucker punch to the gut as well. This particular couple had literally adopted all of their children and I wanted to discuss it with them to learn what I could. In order to feel prepared, I spent a good portion of that day and the day before cleaning my house like a madwoman, which was exhausting. Then I agonized over the menu, made *way* too much food, and went entirely over-the-top in trying to make a perfect presentation. In truth, I was trying to look as if we deserved to be parents somehow. As if the difference in my chicken pot pie coming out perfectly or my baseboards passing the white glove test would be the breaking point in these friends of ours giving us adoption advice. Yep, no crazy there! When it came right down to it though, the dinner was perfectly fine and our friends were very gracious. They were very free with their knowledge and were open to any questions we needed to ask. They shared their various experiences with us, and even brought a few books on open adoption versus closed/private adoption. It was educational and a good first step for me personally to begin embracing adoption as an actual avenue for our family. It was also very difficult. This dinner represented the first time in two years that I had *openly* and *outwardly* acknowledged our potential need for adoption. I mean, I had always been in love with the *idea* of adopting a child, but to truly admit that perhaps adoption was our *only* option was a bigger pill to swallow. This dinner went great, and the company was great, but on the inside I was a ball of nerves. When they finally left, I sighed a big sigh and wept a little on the inside. I felt like closing the door on their visit was somehow closing the door, already, on our last two-week wait. Even though at that point we were only halfway through the wait, I was mentally writing off this last cycle as a failure. I felt as if part of me was dying inside as I watched the final days of our plans for a baby slip out of my grasp.

Finally, with Halloween passed and the dinner done, it was time for my husband to go out of town on his business trip for the week. Coincidentally, this was the same week that would end our final two-week wait and end our infertility journey. He asked me to come with him on the trip; I said no. He asked me to postpone my final blood pregnancy test until he returned; I said no. I did not want to delay the inevitable, and I certainly did not want to be "that wife" that tagged along on her husband's business trips because she had no life. In truth, I knew he would really enjoy the rare opportunity to work face-to-face with his otherwise virtual crew. This trip was a chance for him to get a dose of normal, manly, working time, and be away from this crazy, hormonal existence of late. I did not want to ruin that for him by being a bored, emotional, black hole with my baby worries. No, I felt it was best that he go, and me struggle through this last week on my own. That Monday, we drove him to the airport, hugged and kissed our good-byes, and I went back home and proceeded to plan for my week long redecorating project. I had decided I would pull a *While You Were Out* and completely gut and remodel his office. It had been something I had wanted to do forever and never had the chance. I figured it would be a nice treat for him, and a great way for me to honor all his hard work. Likewise, what a *great* way to keep my mind off the impending deadline of doom that was coming on that Thursday. Nothing like working yourself to death to keep from thinking about a blood test. Yep, no crazy there!

Monday, I purchased paint and paint supplies, and proceeded to remove every piece of furniture, files, computer equipment, etc., out of that room. I did not get much further that first day and I utterly *crashed* exhausted that night as I went to bed. I was glad I had worked hard, since normally I do not sleep well when Kevin's gone, but that night I was ready to drop and did just that. Tuesday, I cleaned the walls, and proceeded to paint all the cutting in work, as well as did a little shopping for the extra "accessories" I needed such as shelves, frames, wall décor, cord control, etc. . Again, I stayed so busy that day that I was utterly exhausted again and my eyes were shut before my head ever hit the pillow. That same routine followed me through Wednesday and each night before bed, Kevin and I would chat on the phone. We would recount our days, and catch up with each other before bedtime. He knew I was up to something, but also knew enough not to press me on the subject. He was *very* careful not to ask how I was feeling, and instead told me loved and missed me and wished he could be there on Thursday for the big blood test. I told him each and every night, truthfully no less, that I was doing well. *And I meant it*! I was staying busy during the days and had been feeling so much better emotionally that it was a relief to work and be occupied. On top of all the remodel work I was doing, I had scheduled our first appointment with an adoption attorney in California for the following Monday, and we had already received our preliminary packet in the mail of info to go over. I was being proactive and getting *so* much stuff done. I was so proud of myself that I even gave myself another mental gold star. I physically felt great and had not thought too much about the Thursday appointment. Any other month, I would have been taking pregnancy tests each and every day, sometimes twice a day, by this point of our two-week wait, but not this month. I was finally starting to accept the end to this road and was ready to just get it over with. I was a little sad at the understanding that I had finally been beat into submission over having *no* children of my own, but I was also grateful to see the trials come to an end. I was ready to move on to a new phase in our lives, and get all this behind me. I felt confident that we had done all we could do... I felt ready to get past the Thursday blood test and on with our lives. Or at least, I *thought* I was ready.

Facing My Fear

Thursday came, and my appointment was set for 8:00 a.m. to give blood for the test and they would call me that afternoon. That morning, I got up, showered, took care of the dogs, and began the drive to Dr. Slater's office. As I pulled out of my garage, I turned on the radio and guess what song was on. Yep, *that song*! That song about praising God through the storms of life, and recognizing that my help comes from the Maker of heaven and earth and how I will lift my eyes up to the Lord. I drove and blasted that song as loud as I could and sang at the top of my lungs and, of course, cried. Cried and cried and prayed to God. By now, you would think my car was my personal therapy session as much crying and praying as I had done in it, but it was the only time I was completely distraction-free! God could *reach me* in my car, I guess. I cried and prayed, but my prayer was different than it had ever been before. I did not beg for a baby this time. Unlike the weeks and months and years that had preceded this moment, I stopped begging and accepted that God already knew my heart's desire. I did not beg God to forgive my wicked past. I did not ask Him to stop punishing my husband for my sins, as if God was a horrible judge sitting on a cloud, smiting people at random. I knew God was not punishing me in that way and I accepted His forgiveness, as He had offered it. Freely. God had died on the cross for my sins, and I had accepted the gift I did not deserve from the one true God who did not deserve the sacrifice He made. My faith had grown so much and I finally understood that it was by God's *grace alone* that I would be saved. Not by my works, or begging prayers, or efforts, but my simple faith. I did not promise God the moon if He would bless us with a child, as if God was some loan shark bargainer. I did not ask over and over for God to open my womb or any of the other things I had done in the past years… He already knew my heart and what I wanted. This time I came, honestly and alone, to God and faced my fears in the mirror of Him. That I was sad and heartbroken by our journey, and that I could not honestly understand why we could not conceive on our own. I still did not understand why He took Peanut from us so soon, and I did not know why He would not bless us again with another child. I admitted that I was unable to carry this burden by myself and did not *want* to anymore. I told God that I did not know what else to do or where else to go and that I needed *Him* to help me through this and to make my heart okay with whatever His plan was. I was brutally honest with God and myself about how I would be devastated to never have my own biological child and to never experience the joys of pregnancy and birth, but that I would honestly and truthfully love any adopted child that God gave us with all my heart. I was equally honest that even in this, I would need God's help. I begged God for sure, but not to make me pregnant. This final time, this last tear-filled and broken prayer, I begged God to make my heart okay with *His* plan. To soften my heart, heal my hurts, and make me a more willing participant in whatever *He* wanted for my life. Or, as a dear friend of mine had well-stated, I was not totally willing yet, but I was willing to be *made* willing.

This heartfelt, brutally honest prayer was the entirety of my thirty minute drive to Dr. Slater's office. I cried the whole way and talked to God. I admitted out loud that I would love and honor Him no matter what, and I would equally love and honor my husband no matter what, but that I needed God's help to be graceful and have courage to let my own will and dreams go. It was the most therapeutic, exhausting, and emotional thirty minute drive I had ever experienced. And considering how many of these drives I had made in the previous years, that was saying something. I felt as if I had rolled down the window to my car and chunked that weight around my neck out the window. I was done lugging that thing around and I was ready to be free from it. By the time I arrived at Dr. Slater's office, I was a puffy, snotty, stopped-up blob of a woman. I pulled into the parking lot, parked the car, noted that I was right on time, and then sat there for a good five minutes. I knew I had to go in, but I could not make myself do it. I could not even find the courage to turn the car off; I could not face what I knew would be the end of the road. This was so final, so finite; there would be no more tries after this. This final negative pregnancy test was somehow so much bigger to me…it was forever. We would not try again and hope some more, we would not pursue more drugs, more tests, more time, we would not even take a few days to enjoy our favorite wines/foods and then hurry-up to jump back into the game. This was the big final checkered flag in our long and hard run race.

I suddenly doubted my husband's request, and my subsequent denial, to postpone the test. At least if he was here with me, he would hold my hand and talk to me and pray with me and be my courage to walk through the door. But he was not there, and I was, alone and red-eyed in the parking lot, trying to psych myself up enough to just get it over with. I decided I could not do it alone so I looked for rein-forcements. I could not get a hold of my husband for some reason, so I called another support person who I felt would fully understand the insanity of my inability to get out of the car…my stepmother. I called her and she chatted with me for a few minutes. I did not go into the whole thirty minute car ride story with her; I did not need to. She asked me what was up, and I simply told her, "I am at the doctor's office and I am in the parking lot and I just don't think I can do this." That was all she needed. She knew what that day was for us... my whole family knew. She knew all that I was *not* saying about how hard it was for me to go in and get that final blood test. I wish now I had written down what she said, because it was perfect. She was the angel I needed at that moment... she was my little life line of guts and courage. It was exactly what I needed to hear—just a small and very loving nudge—to get me out of the car, through the office doors, and into the waiting room.

After that, everything went as expected. They called me back, took the blood, and sent me home to wait for a phone call later that day. The ride home was less emotional, which was good because I had very little left to spend. I did do some more praying, but otherwise went home and proceeded to finish painting my husband's office.

I felt, all in all, that I was as prepared as I possibly could be for this to be over. I had tried my best for the past two years, and what did I have to show for it?

- Innumerable blood, ovulation, and pregnancy tests
- Twenty thousand-plus dollars in medical costs spent out-of-pocket
- Two thousand-plus miles driven to and from various specialists
- Twenty-four consecutive months of Metformin
- Fifteen months of Clomid (the last twelve months consecutively)
- Seven IUIs with sperm washing
- Six different doctors, specialists, and naturalists of some kind (not including nurses)
- Four months of injectable stimulation meds, sono-wands, and trigger shots
- Three minor diagnostic or treatment-related surgeries
- Two-plus solid years of trying to have a baby
- One heartbreaking and life-shaping death
- Zero Babies in my Arms

HEATHER D. NELSON

I could freely admit at this point, that I was done; there was nothing more I could handle. I was beyond blessed to have my marriage as intact as it was, but I knew that it could not withstand this amount of stress and pressure forever without eventually starting to crack. I knew that financially we had gone as far as we could intelligently go. We had worked hard during that first year to get our credit card debts paid off and begin saving up what cash we could, and that paid our way through our second year of treatments. But even with that effort, our savings was drained and any further efforts would require bank loans and other financed options that would have added additional—and unnecessary––stresses to our lives. Physically, I was also at the end of myself. I was exhausted all the time, and the pain and achiness and weariness were just about too much. No more, it was time. All that was left was for me to accept the plan God had for us. All that was left was for me to *let go* and *let God* do with me—with us—what He wanted. From where I was sitting, God did not want us to conceive our own child at this time, He wanted us to pursue adoption or some other avenue, but biological childbearing was clearly not in His plans for us. But again, as was usual in times when I tried to peg exactly what I thought I understood about God and His plan for me, I was dead wrong.

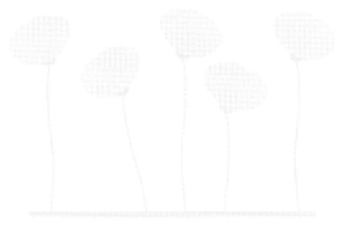

Clearly, God Has Other Plans

On that final Thursday, I went home from Dr. Slater's office (after a perfunctory stop at Starbucks for a little cup of happy) and proceeded to do the final work on Kevin's office. I dove into my husband's office with a vengeance. He would be home on Saturday, and our first appointment with the adoption counselor was that following Monday, and a new leg of our life would begin. I felt I needed to prove to him, or me, or both of us, that I could finish this task on my own. Like finishing this office meant I was ready for adoption or something. Somehow I had equated this office project as being the turning point in our lives and I simply *had* to get it done, in full, before I picked him up at the airport on Saturday. Sure, my back hurt from moving furniture, and I was exhausted from the long hours of painting, hanging, moving, and cleaning, but who cares. I was busy and preparing myself mentally for what was ahead. Do not ask me what crazy pill I was taking to think that painting the walls in that tiny 10 foot by 11 foot room would be the closure I needed, but there you have it, in all my whacked-out glory. After all, why should the crazy, illogical thought train stop now?

I packed up and cleaned up the painting peripherals, and proceeded to hang the final shelves and move the larger pieces of office furniture back into their newly remodeled home. Honestly, I had lost complete track of time when the phone first rang. I nearly jumped out of my skin as I ran to find it buried under the paraphernalia of my insanity. Alas, it was Kevin for the *third* time that day. He had called me several times "checking in." I knew, even though he never asked, that he was as anxious about that blood test as I was. He was trying so hard to play it cool and not make things harder on me, which I loved him for. He was also equally nervous about the results, which I loved him even more for. As always, I told him I was fine and no I had not heard anything yet but I would let him know when I did.

When the phone rang again that afternoon for the fourth time, I honestly expected it to be my husband again. However, my anxiety level was immeasurable when the caller ID said it was Dr. Slater. After jumping near out of my skin, again, I took a deep breath and answered the phone. It was Dr. Slater's office, one of her nurses. I had already prepared my response. Each month the nurses would apologize to us for not having better news and prior to this I would be so wrapped up in my own sadness that I never thought how hard it must be on them to deliver that news. After all, they were in the business of making babies! Surely it must be discouraging to them when their efforts fail. I was determined that this month, I would not breakdown on the phone for whichever poor woman who drew the short straw and had to call me. I was all rehearsed to both tell the nurse that it was *okay* that she did not have better news, and that no, we had no plans to move forward but rather we wanted to take a break for awhile. I was even planning on sounding near chipper with my rehearsed speech so as to reassure her of my positive mental state. I gave myself a mental gold star for being prepared and was actually not at all emotional. I picked up the phone and the conversation went something like this:

"Hello?"
"Is this Heather?"
"Yes it is." I said as I took a deep breath and prepared for my graceful rejection speech

"I have good news for you!" The nurse said cheerily

"That's okay, I was expecting a negative te… *What!?*"

Dr. Slater's nurse giggled as she said, "We have *good* news for you…. you're pregnant!"

"*What?* Are you calling the right patient because if not, that's just mean!"

The nurse sounded nervous now as she asked me, "Is this Heather on Aberdeen Avenue with DOB of May…, and a S.S.N. of…?"

"Yes, that's me. What the…"

"Then yes," she sighed with relief, "I'm calling the right person. You are pregnant!"

"Are you sure?"

The nurse giggled again. "Yes, we're sure."

Dumbfounded, I asked, "How pregnant? What was the beta number?"

"Your number was one hundred sixty-six, and anything over fifteen is considered positive."

As I picked, my jaw up off the floor I said, "So then that's like really, *really* pregnant? "

"Yep, you are really, totally, completely, 100 percent pregnant." She was full on laughing at me at this point.

The rest of the conversation was an abbreviated set of instructions from the nurse on what I should do and should not do. She mentioned I should keep taking my progesterone supplements until we hit nine weeks, and that in the meantime I should avoid lunch meats, soft cheeses, and heavy lifting. I looked around the partially put together office and sort of laughed to myself about that last one. We ended the call with her scheduling our first OB ultrasound and checkup, and as I hung up the phone, I sat there utterly stunned speechless. I stared at the newly painted walls, which suddenly looked like baby nursery blue to me. The furniture that was incomplete in its placement suddenly took on a deeper meaning. This was not merely office furniture, I thought, this is a *daddy's office furniture*! I think I stared at the floor for a good five minutes trying to process what this meant. It was just not fully sinking in.

Here I was, all prepared for a negative pregnancy test. We had tried for years, and spent an incredible amount of time, effort, money, emotion, stress, and worry with trying to conceive and I had finally accepted that the end was most definitely nigh. I was even prepared with a speech to accept the bad news and make the *nurse* feel better about delivering it. I was really truly completely unsure what to think about this news. My mind sort of shut down as I envisioned, *tentatively*, my new due date, what our baby would look like, and what our lives would be like with a little one crawling around. My heart, still not mended from the acceptance of being childless, was now reeling in the idea that maybe, just maybe, adoption would not be our *only* option. I'm not sure how long I sat there, but at some point, one of my dogs walked over and nudged my hand for a quick pat on the head and she had such a happy look on her face, as if she knew. I started to laugh out loud, then my mind started racing of all the things I had to do and how would I tell my husband and… and… *and…*

As I sat there, in shock, laughing like a crazy person and talking to my dog and wondering what to do next, my husband, with his mother's flare for fortuitous timing, called. I answered a bit *too* quickly, but schooled myself to not say anything at that time. I know that sounds awful, but it was true. I was not prepared to tell him yet. Aside from not yet having had time to process it myself, I had already started culminating a plan on how to spring it on him when he arrived home on Saturday, and I did not want to spoil my chance to give him the shock of a lifetime. He had *earned* the wonderful surprise as much as I had, if not more. I wanted to make it perfect for him. He asked how I was doing, I said fine. He asked what I was doing, I said I was finishing up my little project. He told me about his day thus far and made small talk that he normally hates to make. When I was not more forthcoming, he finally broke down and asked me point-blank if I had heard from the doctor yet. I took a deep breath, and said in my most calm and level voice possible, "Honey, I wish I could tell you good news, but I can't." *Which was partially true,* I did *wish* I could tell him good news. Him and every person I had *ever* met in fact, but I wanted to wait a little bit and process things. He blessedly did not push the subject and moved on.

We chatted and small talked a little more, and then hung up the phone just before I nearly cracked and told him the whole story. I felt more than a little guilty for misleading him, but also a little proud of myself for containing *the secret of the century*. I now knew exactly what to do for him though, and that helped justify my secrecy a little more.

Finishing Touches

As it happened, I was nearly finished with the office remodel and only needed to put the final finishing touches and get the rest of the furniture moved in, etc. I was instantly paranoid about moving the furniture, as if moving the desk *now* would make a difference from moving it two hours prior to that call. But who can argue with the insanity at this point?

I called up Pastor Jeff, who had been praying and counseling us all this time, and asked if he could help me move the furniture back *into* the office that I had moved *out*. He immediately said he would gladly help, and then paused and asked, "How come you cannot move it back in if you moved it out though?" I hesitated and then said, "Well, I moved it out earlier this week before I found out, just today, that I'm pregnant and I'm not supposed to do any heavy lifting." He paused for a minute and then blurted out, "Whoa, back up. This is much bigger news. *Heather*, you're Pregnant? " I told the story to him of my conversation with the nurse, and then told him of how I was trying to *surprise* Kevin before he came home, so Jeff had to keep it under his hat. He was clearly excited, and promised that he and his lovely wife would be in fervent prayer for us all during these early weeks.

After that call, I left my house and immediately went down to a little boutique shop near our house that sold all manner of home décor items. You know the kind. It was an eclectic little decorative place full of what-nots that are oh-so-lovely and change out by the season and always keep you coming in to shop and browse some more. Well, as it happened, this little shop also did custom signs made-to-order of any phrase/saying you wanted. I walked in at around 6:00 p.m. on Thursday night and was near *bursting* with excitement to describe what I wanted.

For the record, in case you did not know already, I'm *horrible* about keeping secrets of my own when I'm excited and happy about them.

Keeping secrets of other people is easy, but if I'm excited about something personal, it practically oozes out of my pores! As such, when the lady asked if she could help me, it was with no small amount of restraint that I calmly stated, "I was wondering about your custom sign services. I have something specific in mind and would really love to have it done by Saturday morning if at all possible." Oh the mental restraint it took to *not* yell from the top of my lungs that I was pregnant was astounding. The woman, and subsequently the owner, was very sweet and said that she would love to do the sign, but that she could not turn it around that fast because they were busy swapping out their inventory for the holidays that evening and there would be no time. I definitely understood, but expressed my disappointment in that I was hoping to complete my husband's surprise. She then asked, "Oh, what surprise are you planning?" *This*, of course, was my opening to tell her about the *entire* two-year struggle, the surprise positive results, the office remodel, and my infamous "sign" idea in twenty words or less! She was so wrapped up in my story, and was clearly excited for me, that she then said, "Oh goodness, well that's just too big a surprise and I cannot let you go without this sign, so yes, I'll call my husband right now and have him start cutting the wood. Let's pick your fonts and wording and get this sign made." I do not recall exactly, but I might have hugged her at this point! Everything was coming together well and I could not contain myself with the excitement of it all.

After the sign was ordered, I went home, ate some dinner, and sat there, marveling at how different my world suddenly was and wondering about what my husband's response would be to all this. Needless to say, I got *very little* sleep that night, but as I laid my head on my pillow, you *know* I was doing some *fervent* praying!

Friday was a bit of a blur. Pastor Jeff came over and finished moving the furniture for me, while I got the last of the shelves hung and picture frames on the wall and such. I cleaned up the last of the remodel "junk" and vacuumed, and then took a step back and looked at my handiwork. All in all, I was pleased with the results. The office was cool and friendly

HEATHER D. NELSON

and relaxing in color. The junk I removed created more space, and the shelving I hung both on the walls and in the closet created much more usable space and organization. The sheer aspect of *dusting* all those electronic elements made things more clean and refreshing feeling, and now all I needed was the finishing touches. I showered and headed out for my afternoon errands.

First on my agenda was to get my nails done. I was *particularly* excited about this one too. My nail lady, Deb, and the nice older woman who always had her appointment before mine, Kay, had been keeping close tabs on all our baby-making efforts over the past year. Besides, where I come from hairdressers and nail techs are family and counselors wrapped up in one. I knew, without a doubt, they would ask about my pregnancy test, and I was silently rehearsing my response to them. Sure enough, I walked in and stood there as Deb and Kay and the other hair techs chatted. Suddenly, Selma (the hairdresser at the next station over who had also been keeping tabs on us) looked at me without any prompting and said, "Oh my goodness, you're pregnant." *Just like that*! To which I immediately confirmed, and the whole room started "ooohing" and "aaahing" and squealing over my news. I told the story of the doctor's call, and by the time I was done, Selma, Tara, Deb, Kay and some other woman I had never met knew we were expecting. I was thrilled to share the news with them and they were equally thrilled to hear it. Sharing this news with Deb and the gang was fantastic for me. And Kay, the other nail client, immediately started referring to herself as Auntie Kay and was *thrilled* for me.

This now made seven people who I had managed to blab this secret to *before* my husband. There was a part of me that felt guilty about this, but an equal part of me that so wanted to present the surprise to him in a special way. I felt he had earned it and I did not want to deny him the excitement of "figuring it out" when he saw the office and the special sign I had made.

After my nails were done and I was fawned over by all the ladies for nearly an hour, I glowed my way to my car and headed over to a local department store that had a baby department in it. Once there, I went up and down every aisle arguing with myself that I should not buy anything until we were into our second trimester, *and* that I *should* get a few things to increase my husband's surprise. They had little socks that said "I 'heart' Daddy," and I had to get those. They also had this book for fathers-to-be... yep, got that too.

About the time I was restraining myself from purchasing baby's first laptop computer, my own mother called me out of the blue to *check in*. Remember, my mother always knew *when* we were testing for pregnancy, but vowed to *never* call and dig about it, assuming that if I did not call her it must be negative. Well this cycle, she called to chit-chat and I knew this was her way of "fishing" for the pregnancy test results. After debating about not answering my phone for a millisecond, I decided I simply had to answer her call, but I *would* keep it a secret. *I would, I would, I would!* We chatted about this and that and I could tell she was being subtle, but wanting to know if we were pregnant or not. I kept telling myself that if I just kept my mouth shut, she'd never know and then I could tell her with the rest of the family at a later date that Kevin and I mutually decided on. But no, the excitement was too much. Before I exploded all over the store, I decided it best to cave and tell the news to her. Kicker was, she was in the car with my aunt and she had to promise both to *not* react at all and *not* tell. I am not sure how her own head did not explode when I told her she had another grandbaby on the way. And yeah, that was *one more person* I "leaked" my surprise to. I am not sure how my husband did not find out all the way in Tennessee at this point, considering the news now reached all the way to Dallas, Texas and back. I was officially the world's WORST secret keeper but I did not care. I was also now saddled with a new label–***expectant mother***.

The Big Reveal

Finally, mercifully, Saturday arrived. I was beyond excited to pick Kevin up from the airport and I thought I would burst. As I drove to the airport, speeding only a little, I rehearsed all the ways I would make small talk and *not* burst with excitement. *This* was the hard part; this was that final stretch. I had to both pick him up and not tell him right then and there, but also make it *all* the way home for his surprise office remodel and let him discover the big secret on his own. And let's face it, this secret was not being kept well to begin with, so my hopes were not great that I could pull this off!

Sure enough, I managed to pick him up at the airport without any little slips. I was afraid he would take one look at my face and see right through my very thinly veiled level of excitement, but he did not. We made with the chit-chat, grabbed luggage, and spent the drive home discussing his trip, the work, the travel, etc., which was funny to me, because we discussed all these same things in smaller measurements each night before bed while he was away, but whatever. At this point, I was clinging on to whatever I could for dear life to try and maintain my calm.

As we pulled into the garage of our house, I really thought for sure I would combust with the restraint. It took every ounce of God-given strength I had in me to calmly help him get the luggage from the car and enter the house. I set my purse and keys in their normal spot, and resisted the urge to bolt, like lightning, straight to the office. Of course, my husband knew that I was working on some massive project, so he immediately started looking around. When he got to his office, he flipped on the light and stuck his head in the office and said, "Wow, you painted and rearranged furniture and hung a little sign over the window. I like it honey, it looks really nice. Thanks," and he gave me a hug. My jaw hit the floor.

Wow, you *painted*? *Thanks*? *REALLY?!?!*

I about fell over. *This* was my big moment, the week of remodeling and rearranging and planning and scheming and the *giant sign* I had painstakingly purchased and hung to make the final announcement, and he completely missed it—missed the whole thing. Now I will grant that my husband really was not the most observant of people when it came to subtle things, but *seriously*, I was to the point of a breakdown right then and there. I mentally contained myself and calmly said to him, "Honey, you cannot get the full effect if you do not go all the way *in* the office and fully look around." So with my extra nudging, he went all the way *in* the office, stood in the middle of the room, slowly turned a complete three-sixty, and commented all the way around as he turned. "No really, I like what you did. The pictures on the walls, the shelves holding my computer and books and stuff. I like where you put the printer and the extra desktop space will be nice, and that sign that says "Daddy's Office," it all looks really great. I can tell you worked hard." That was it... *again?!?* At this point my patience was shot and I was wound tighter than a spring. I looked at him and said, "Honey, *seriously?* You don't get it?" He looked at me with a confounded expression, so I continued, "We're pregnant."

Dramatic pause of earth-shattering silence.

"We are?" he asked, "Are you sure?" At that point, he looked around again and finally the pieces fell together. I could see the lightbulb go on behind his eyes as he saw, for the first time, the picture frame that said "Baby" in it, the little socks that said "I 'heart' Daddy," and the cigar next to his monitor. Finally, he noted the *Daily Inspiration for Fathers* book on the shelf next to the *Baby Names* and *Father-To-Be* books. Finally, he recognized the sign, the large *white* sign with black lettering that said, "Daddy's Office," and you could see the click when the final piece fell into place. He looked at me and laughed and I laughed and we hugged, and cried. I explained the past three days to him and how I wanted so much to surprise him, but it was hard to keep the secret. He admitted that he had been hoping all along, and that when I did not come right out and say the test was negative on the phone, that he immediately told his coworkers in Tennessee that he was hoping and praying that this was it, but did not want to say that to me and get my hopes up if he was wrong. We both laughed some more and cried and hugged some more, and I have no idea how the rest of that evening went, since I was so strung out and emotional that it is a complete blur to me. A blissful, happy, terrifying, wondrous, unplanned, unexpected blur. But I do remember one thing.

We prayed.

Right then and there in the office, we prayed and thanked God for this beautiful, precious gift He gave to us, this blessing, *this* miracle. We thanked Him, and asked that He protect the baby and me over the coming months, that we could both remain healthy and strong. This was the best and most surprising prayer I think we had ever done together as a couple.

The weekend of Kevin's arrival was marked with several more memorable moments. We talked about waiting to tell everyone of our news until we were into the second trimester, but that was harder than it appeared. That night after dinner, we agreed to at least tell our parents. After all, my mother knew, and I felt guilty not telling his mother, who was tracking my ovulation almost as closely as I was. Then, that Sunday at church, we had two different couples that knew us so well that they literally figured it out without us even telling them. We figured at that point that our attempts to hide this were going to be far more difficult than even we realized. After all, we already had two years, three states, and an entire congregation of our church praying for us to have a baby––it made sense that they would occasionally ask how things were, and you *know* I was not going to be able to lie about this good news. And why would we want to—we were euphoric. Shocked beyond measure that after all this time, and preparations of our hearts for ending this road to family-hood, it would finally happen this way for us, but still blissfully happy. Happy and nervous. We had been pregnant before and had suffered dearly with the heartbreaking loss of Peanut. We had spent over a year of trying with doctors and specialists and sadly, were so overeducated on what it took to get pregnant, that we knew exactly how fragile and frail this miracle of ours was. And we knew, knew to our very core, how quickly this joyous time could turn for the worse. So we prayed *daily*. Prayed to God thanking him for this miracle, this blessing, and thanked him for giving us this opportunity once again. We also prayed for strength and courage, mainly for me. Courage to not worry, courage to let God lead us in this pregnancy. We prayed each day, sometimes multiple times a day, that the baby would be strong and healthy and growing as it should be. And through all the prayer and happy apprehension, was a looming appointment that we had made and I felt we needed to keep.

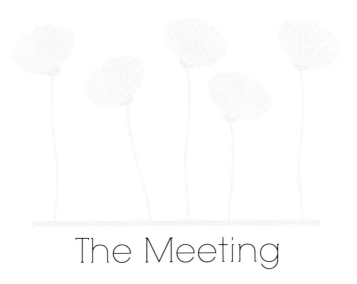

The Meeting

Midway through the two-week wait before our pregnancy test, and before Kevin even left for his business trip, I had scheduled an appointment with an adoption attorney. I was, after all, convinced that we would fail this cycle too, and was doing what I normally do in emotionally tense situations: plan, organize, prepare, and imitate control!

As such, the appointment had been set for almost two full weeks, and we had already received the initial packet of information. But after finding out that we were in fact pregnant, we were torn. Should we cancel the consult and throw this blessing in God's face if, in fact, He *wanted* us to adopt, and our *big, fat, positive pregnancy test* was His way of gifting us for obeying his will, or should we move forward with the adoption and risk getting multiple babies at the same time, both naturally and via adoption? And what of the money concerns of adoption costs mixed with prenatal care? And did we even qualify for adoption now? And of course, there was that fear way back in my mind that what if we passed over this adoption opportunity, only to miscarry yet another baby and be back at square one? Would we move forward with adoption then, or use this pregnancy as another sign for hope to keep trying? And if we kept trying would it be another two years of physical torture and financial drain and emotional havoc and if so, could I withstand that? The questions in my head were multiplying almost as rapidly as I could form coherent thoughts and, of course, all of it underlying the current of being happy and fearful of this pregnancy at the same time. If I had thought for one second that ending our infertility struggle would relieve all my worry and stress, I was sorely mistaken.

After thinking things over for a day or two, I decided to voice my concerns to my husband. I even agreed with that still small voice in my head that reminded me this was *his* journey too, and not only my call to make. Finally, whattya know, that little voice and I were on the same page! I explained all my convoluted thinking to Kevin and he, in his inexplicable way, was able to follow my crazed train of multi-thought. He fully supported my decision in the end. I felt we should honor our commitment to the adoption consultation at the very least, and then see where we are led at that point, and he agreed. So with that decision made, at 1:00 p.m. on Monday, a mere four days after the positive test and only two days after the big office reveal, the adoption attorney called us from out-of-state and we began our phone interview.

The meeting started cordially enough with introductions all around, and then she began giving us lots of information. The process, the norms, the surprises, what we need to do now versus later, what they do, etc., etc., etc. I took dutiful notes and we asked plenty of questions along the way. All in all, the woman was very helpful and informative, but in the back of my mind was still that nagging question: *Should we be doing this or not?* I was beginning to worry that we would not have closure after this meeting like I was hoping for. Then what would we do?

Finally, toward the end, we start talking about cost. Now of course, my darling husband began his own note taking at this point, but in reality there was little she could tell us. Each state had their own rules and each adoption scenario was mildly different from every other one and there were multiple options, yada, yada, yada. She asked if I had gone through the packet she mailed to me and that was my opening. I said, "Well, honestly, we received the packet, but then my husband was called away on business last week, and then we received the good news that we are expecting a baby too now, and we have not had a chance since then to really delve into the details yet, much less determine what comes next. And frankly, I was not sure if our own pregnancy would put us out of the running for an adoption or not, so I was going to ask you at this meeting."

Her response, I believe, was a message direct from God. As I stopped rambling and we sat there listening to the phone on baited breath, she calmly asked if this was our first pregnancy. Kevin told her that we had been pregnant before, but had miscarried, and I then chimed in that we had struggled for nearly two-plus years to get here and were not sure we could even become pregnant again until now. I felt fairly confident we were supplying way too much information to her, and surely she would get uncomfortable talking to us, but she did not skip a beat. She then asked if there was any reason to believe I would not carry this baby to term. That caught me off guard a little. I was not expecting to discuss the "permanence" of my baby with her, but when I thought it over I realized for the first time that we had *no reason*. We were never told that Peanut's loss was anything other than an unfortunate circumstance. There was no chromosomal or genetic issue with the baby then, and we never found anything chronic with me to believe I could not carry to term. I said, "Well, no. They sent things off for testing, but never found any definitive cause for the previous miscarriage either with me or the baby, so no, not that we know of."

At that point, this lovely woman, who had never met us before, who had not ever expressed if she was Christian or not, nor had asked if we were, then said,

> I think God has given you *your* baby already that you are carrying. Adoption is very stressful and taxing, and this is a time for you to just relax and enjoy. So my advice is to put all our paperwork up in a closet. Away for now, and simply focus on *your* baby and being healthy and stress-free. If something happens in the future and you feel differently, you know how to find me and we can pick this conversation up right where we left off, but for now, relax and enjoy this time with your husband and *the baby God gave you.*

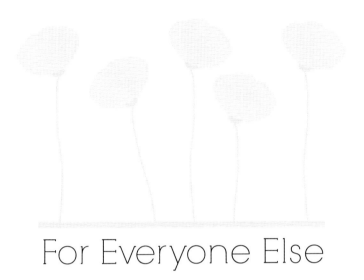

For Everyone Else

At this point, honestly, I was unsure how to move forward on this book. Sure, I had told our story in all its gruesome glory, and I could put, "… and they lived all the live long day" at the end and call it done. But had I accomplished all I wanted? Had I done what I set out to do, which was to give a book to the world of married couples that could not only make them feel less alone in their struggles, but also help encourage them, guide them a little, and hopefully spare them a small modicum of the isolation and pain that we felt. In truth, had I left out this next portion, the answer to all the above would be "No."

Our story, while an interesting read (hopefully), is really only a part of what I wanted to share. The other part was more of a guide to maneuvering the very rocky waters of infertility and pregnancy loss. But not so much a "self-help" type guide, as rather a "Wow, I wish someone had written this for us" type section. There are many things that I learned about myself, my husband, our marriage, our friends, our family, our church, our faith, and more. They were rocky lessons and hard-learned, and I often wished there was some kind of road map out there to give me some advice on *how* to proceed. What to take seriously, and what to blow off and ignore. I wished there were little Post-Its I could print off somewhere and anonymously hand out to my friends and family to tell them the things to say or not say. And moreover, I wanted someone out there that could truly understand our situation, feel our pain, and give us a little hope that the road we were on was not only noble and right and good, but also well worth the walk, and one walked with friends at our side.

So this final chapter, of this very long-winded and hopefully inspiring, if not at the very least worth a laugh book, is dedicated to that cause. And hopefully, some poor, struggling couple will be browsing the shelves of their favorite book store and see our cover and think to themselves, "Finally, something for *us.*" For those couples in the trenches right now, flip to the epilogue for advice geared to you. But first, let me address some information for everyone else. You know who you are, the friend or family member who has never struggled with infertility or pregnancy loss, but knows someone who is. *This* particular section is for you.

Things Better Left Unsaid

Ask any couple out there who has struggled with infertility what the most hated phrase of their life is and they'll almost all reply, with a vehement glare of anger in their eyes, "Just relax." It's by far the most favored and easily leaned on platitude that other fertile and well-meaning people spout off as supposed helpful advice. In truth though, it is not the only phrase or intention that is commonly repeated and, in fact, it is not even the most painful. Undoubtedly, the people making these statements feel that they *are* helping and have *no clue* how cutting and hurtful these things can be received. When you get down to the heart of things, lack of experience and proper education can make even the most well-meaning and loving person *seem* hurtful. What's that phrase about the road to hell being paved with good intentions? It is certainly true here. What many people perceive as helpful, or even inspiring, can cut like a knife to the heart of a couple who was told they have a slim and none chance of conceiving, or worse yet have just lost a child. And the sad part is, no one *means* to be hurtful. No one intentionally plans ahead with their list of hurtful statements, to make sure they give that poor couple one more reason to cry or be angry. All these sayings are rooted in good intentions and truly intended to try and ease some pain or, if nothing else, help us all feel less alone.

As such, I figured it would be helpful to compile a list of the most common phrases I heard during our journey and try to educate the fertile world. Moreover, I wanted to take that list and explain both why it is intended to be helpful (for those couples on the receiving end of these statements) and why it is a hurtful, and sometimes irresponsible, statement to make (for those of you who have these phrases in your repertoire, but do not know when to use them or when not to use them). So without further ado, below is my list.

Just Relax

This is, by far, one of the most frequently used platitudes that couples trying to conceive hear. Whether they are struggling with infertility or not, *inevitably*, if a couple announces they are "trying," someone will pipe up with "just relax and then it'll happen." Truth be told, there is wisdom in this thought, and it is laced with the best of intentions. In this day and age, where life is rushed and busy and young couples are hurried into buying a house, having kids, getting jobs, etc., etc., there is *great* wisdom in being told that family planning should not be rushed into. Furthermore, many medical doctors will not even evaluate whether or not you are dealing with underlying medical/fertility issues until you have been trying a minimum of eight months or a year, and in that time, many minor issues will have worked themselves out.

For any couple newly married and starting out on the road to parenthood, relaxing is good advice in the beginning. It could be a great time of togetherness as a couple and enjoying each other at new levels and with new perspectives. However, for a couple that is knowingly struggling or has just miscarried a child, this phrase can be unendingly hurtful for many reasons. Namely being, that it can carry the implication that their stress (or lack of relaxation) is in fact *causing* their problems. You see, when a couple first realizes that something is askew in baby-making-ville, the medical doctors immediately put them through a whole slew of tests and begin educating them on all the possibilities that could be factoring into their particular brand of infertility or miscarriage. And when I say "all possibilities," I mean it. Couples are asked to look at things like family/genetic history, personal health history, sexual background, health and nutrition, work and life styles, types of underwear worn, sports played in adolescent years, and more. The result of all this is a couple that is not only very educated, but also a bit paranoid about any and every possible permutation of what *they* may or may not have done to have *caused* this problem. Thus, when some well-meaning and loving person comes along, hears they are struggling, and says "Oh, just relax, that's when it will happen," many couples take their stress level and add that to the menagerie of things that they could be doing *wrong* to thus hinder their family planning. If it sounds crazy to think that way, I assure you, it is a well-earned insanity.

What's more, many couples actually visiting with specialists and dealing with infertility issues have already been trying for quite a long time and are already aware of legitimate medical issues. As such, relaxation *really* is not a factor. They are not being impatient and wanting their way right now, they are really struggling physically, emotionally, and likely financially at this point. Some well-meaning person telling them to relax is, in essence, discounting all that they are going through. It is the equivalent, at times, as saying, "Geez, you're so dramatic. What's your problem? You're fine and you do not need a baby right now." I personally was often able to laugh this comment off, but many couples are very hurt by the fact that someone could actually learn of their struggles and then dismiss them as something so trivial as a stress-induced hindrance. If you know a couple who is trying to conceive and they express concern or impatience at the process, you could ask how long they've been trying, or even if they have reason to be worried. But if there was ever one phrase I would remove from the English language on behalf of all conceiving couples out there, "Just Relax" would be the one I would pick.

Maybe God Doesn't Want This for You

In my understanding, the intent here is to help a couple see that God does have *some* plan for them, and perhaps having a child in this way, or at this time, is not in His plan right now. Not to say it will not happen eventually, just perhaps not in the manner we think is best. Or better yet, perhaps we are being denied what we *think* we want, for some greater blessing that God has in mind for us that we cannot see yet. That one day, we will look back on all our struggles and be able to say, with a smile, that we are so glad God denied us this. Unfortunately, the logic is flawed here on multiple levels.

This was probably the one phrase that hurt me the most during our efforts. It was said to me shortly after our loss of Peanut, and just as we were really beginning our road of options for making a family of our own. We were very educated on all the choices we had to make, and had resigned ourselves to a path of our choosing. When this was said to me personally, admittedly, my first reaction was less than graceful. In fact, I think the thought that went through my mind was, "Gee, thanks. God thinks I would be *such* a bad mother He must divinely sterilize me, or better yet, He thinks the pre-teen mother who puts her baby in the trash can is somehow more deserving of this than me. That's great." Talk about graceless thoughts, huh? It was definitely not one of my shining moments. But in reality, what hurt me the most was that I felt that this person was trying to tell me what they thought God wanted in my life, and that by trying as hard as I was, I was somehow being disobedient. The assumption here being that, a). this person *knew* what God wanted, and b). I had already gone *so far* in my efforts that I should now just give up before going beyond God's will.

Truth be told, no man on earth can truly know the will of God. Does God have a plan for each of us? Absolutely. But are any of us ever all-knowing enough to know the plan for our own life, much less the life of others? Eh, not so much. True infertility is a medical diagnosis. There is something medically non-functioning in one or both of the couple involved that is outside the normal healthy parameters of what should be happening. The same could be said of a heart patient in need of a pacemaker or a diabetic, whose body does not produce enough insulin. If someone seeks medical assistance to remedy their clogged arteries, it is not looked upon as strongly as somehow disobeying God's will or going beyond what God wants for them. And yet, if a couple is told that the woman does not ovulate, or that the man has a sperm production issue due to a physical malformation of his equipment, they are often expected to blindly accept this as the path for their life and not seek any medical intervention whatsoever. I am admittedly trying to tread lightly here, as this is a touchy issue of great debate, but the truth of the matter is that infertility is often far more physically reaching than some people realize. For example, on the surface, a woman might not ovulate and thus, cannot conceive. People might say, "Oh, pray and accept that you cannot have kids," and expect her to move on. But in truth, she's not ovulating because her body has a high resistance to insulin, which is causing a whole slew of other systemic health concerns that do need to be addressed (as is the case for many women suffering from Polycystic Ovarian Syndrome, such as myself). Had I *not* pursued having a baby, I would not have been properly diagnosed with PCOS, and thus been educated and treated for the long-term effects of insulin resistance to my heart and other vital organs.

A couple whose heart yearns for a child does not have any main line into understanding God's will for them anymore than the next person does. But they do have a great desire in their heart to conceive and carry and love and raise a baby. They have very passionate feelings and as such, are often inclined to feel as if they have done all they can feasibly do within their power before letting that dream go. Expecting them to "accept the inevitable" is perhaps something better left between them and God, and not from an outside perspective.

Why Aren't You Just Doing IVF or Adopting

This is one of the more harmless statements, but still one that I heard often. The thought here is to support the couple and ask them about pursuing either one option or another and in so doing make things *easier* on themselves. Adoption, being one extreme, of giving up on conceiving on their own, and IVF, being the opposite extreme, of seeking major medical intervention to help further conception efforts. On the surface, this is a relatively harmless statement to make and can, for many couples, be the welcomed invitation to discuss the thoughts they have had on these topics, one way or another. But as is often the case for many issues raised in this book, emotions run high and can often lead to hurt feelings if not approached delicately.

For example, IVF has become a very popular topic of discussion; given the heightened media attention we have seen lately. To someone who has never had to sit with a reproductive endocrinologist and discuss the options, IVF could be a popular buzz word that is a seeming "fix all" to a couple's conception struggles. In truth, however, IVF is *very* expensive and physically trying. Depending on the level of intervention needed, IVF can run as much as twenty thousand dollars or more *per cycle,* and the odds are not 100 percent guaranteed. To a couple trying to have a baby, it is a daunting number to take in. Moreover, IVF is one of the most medically-intensive treatments out there. Women have to undergo a slew of shots, pills, antibiotics, sonograms, invasive exams, egg retrieval surgeries, implantation, and more. And with all that medical intervention, all they are guaranteed is great cost and poor odds of conception.

IVF is only *one* in a whole menagerie of treatment options available to couples these days. Treatments can start in the very simplistic vitamin/pill regimen, all the way up to IVF/ICSI options, and about one hundred different variations in between. Not to mention the fact that IVF eliminates pretty much *any* real involvement in physical conception from a traditional standpoint. The eggs are actually fertilized *outside* the body and then *re*-implanted. This is often a line that many couples are not morally prepared to cross yet. Moreover, if there are too many eggs to implant at once, they have to decide what to do with their other frozen babies. While a couple may well need IVF in the end, it is a personal decision for them to make and one that likely will take much time, prayer, discussion, and planning for what path will get them to that point. To off-handedly ask why they are not *just* doing IVF could be perceived as you thinking that it is an "easy fix," and that they are silly for avoiding the inevitable.

Adoption is often similarly treated as a quick fix to infertile couples. In reality, it is not an insta-family-cure-all, and can also have multiple paths to get there as well. I know when I personally began researching adoption, I was overwhelmed by the options, cost, restrictions, regulations, timetables, and more. I was both impressed with how cautious agencies were to ensure children were placed in good homes, but also a bit put off by how *difficult* and expensive it can often be for a good couple to actually get the baby they so badly desire. For the couple struggling with their own conception problems, adoption has another layer of emotions piled on top of it. Adoption is often a very slow moving and financially burdensome process. Infertility treatments are very expensive and often very non-timely processes as well. More often than not, a couple has to make a decision to either try adoption *or* try fertility treatments. Very rarely do you see couples that can afford to do both and hope to strike pay dirt one way or another. To a couple who dreams of having their own biological child, adoption is definitely a solution, but a bittersweet one at that. Yes, it is true, a successful adoption would give them a child to love and raise and care for, but they would need to have time to mourn the loss of the child they had dreamed of; the child that had daddy's eyes and mommy's hair. They would lose that precious opportunity to experience pregnancy and birth together as a couple, and would need to put those dreams to rest. Adoption is a wonderful opportunity, both for the family adopting and the child in need of a loving home, but it is not always a quick Band-Aid solution for any couple who is struggling to conceive. Asking a couple why they "do not *just* adopt" is often horribly received as you discounting the greatest of their heart's desires.

In both of these cases, and in many others (surrogacy, surgeries, fostering, etc.), it is better to err slightly on the side of caution. Friends and family *want* to be supportive, but these are heart-wrenching decisions for a couple to make. With a couple struggling for a family, there is *always* more going on under the surface than most people ever know. And sometimes, as was our case, one spouse might want to choose a route that the other spouse is not ready for…and there could already be some marital tension that you are unaware of. While a couple may end up adopting, trying IVF, becoming state foster parents, or using a surrogate, it is not always your place to *suggest* one of these options to them. Instead, you could ask, "What options are you looking at right now?" and then let them share their feelings with you as they see fit.

Or better yet, tell them, "Whatever you decide, I am here for you if you want to talk." When they are ready, they will share what they have decided with the world. Until then, be cautious that you do not add undo pressure toward options that they may not be ready to consider yet or have already ruled out.

The Miscarriage Is God's Way
of Taking Care of Something That Was Wrong

The thought process behind this statement is always to try and find the silver lining in the sadness of a pregnancy loss. Or rather, to find solace and comfort in the reasoning behind something that otherwise has little rhyme or reason to it. As by understanding the "why" of it, one can help to heal the hurt. Another common one in this circumstance is, "Well, at least you know you *can* get pregnant and it will happen again." But in truth, to a couple who just lost a child, these statements offer little by way of comfort, and often dole out a bit of pain that is not intended in the process.

To understand why these statements hurt so much, you must understand the full picture. As my own story has shown, when a couple discovers they are pregnant, they often begin planning and dreaming of what that baby will look like. They discuss the baby's needs, and start preparing their home and life to welcome the new bundle of joy. Beyond that, they may even look long-term at what their baby will be like. What kind of personality will the baby have, and will the baby grow to like music or sports or be an intellect? Some couples, as we did, will even name their baby. In lieu of calling the baby "it," they see that beautiful first sonogram and decide that the baby will have a name. For us, it was Peanut. Our Peanut was the most beautiful gray blob on a screen we had ever seen in our lives to that point, and we would address the baby as Peanut anytime we discussed the pregnancy, both to each other and to our friends and family. As you can imagine, all this increases the attachment to the unborn child and makes the pregnancy *more* special and magical in the minds of those expecting parents.

Now, take all that hope and excitement and anticipation and dreaming and toss on a big dose of cold reality when they discover that the baby is gone. Either through dramatic, painful, messy, emergency-room-trip-worthy cramping, or through a shocking sonogram with no heartbeat followed by heart-wrenching choices; Discovering your baby is suddenly dead is a ton of bricks like no other. The initial shock is only the moments it takes for the reality to set in, but then the real pain comes. They did not lose "it" or "a fetus" or "a pregnancy." They lost a child, *their child.* That couple lost an entire lifetime. The child with daddy's eyes, mommy's hair, musical talent, and a sense of humor will no longer exist. They lost their Peanut, or Bean, or Tadpole. They lost an *entire life* of dreams and hopes that they had planned. They lost the nursery they had planned, and perhaps already started. They lost the excitement of watching the mother's body change and grow. They will never feel the baby move, or see it kick on a sonogram. They will never get those showers celebrating that little life, or get the joy of holding that baby in the delivery room with family by their side, as you revel in the miracle God granted. To the couple who lost the pregnancy, that was their whole world that has been violently ripped from their hearts without their consent, without their knowing, and with no control of the situation. It is a grief that is special and unique. It is a horrible club that you never want to be in, but once there, you immediately recognize the new members. And for those couples struggling, the thought that perhaps the miscarriage was God's way of taking care of an incomplete or incorrect fetus is of *absolutely no* comfort.

Once I learned about what all goes on during the first nine or ten weeks of a pregnancy, it became easier to understand how fragile a pregnancy can be. When we had our miscarriage, Dr. Hayes told us that 75 percent of all first pregnancies end in miscarriage. During those first nine weeks of crucial developing, the baby lays the groundwork of the brain, nervous system, heart, and more. So much has to happen correctly and quickly. Many couples do not even *know* they are pregnant much before the nine week mark, and if something goes wrong, they believe it is a heavy cycle that was a little late. Other couples find out relatively soon after discovering their pregnancy with heavy bleeding and cramping. The rest have what was described as a "missed miscarriage" where you carry the baby for weeks not knowing it's gone. As

HEATHER D. NELSON

Dr. Hayes explained to us, even if we *knew* what was going to happen before it happened, there is little to nothing that could have been medically done in the first trimester to stop a miscarriage. It truly is "one of those things" that happens and cannot always be explained.

Knowing what I know now, I believe miscarriage truly can be God's way of saving the couple more pain later on when a pregnancy is no longer viable. However, that said, when a couple first divulges that they have miscarried, this comment is better saved to a later time, or not said at all. They are grieving in a very personal and unique way. They have lost hopes and dreams, and there are *no* good platitudes to find solace in at that moment. They need to discuss important things like how to grieve and remember the baby (an important step for some couples, not to others). They need to discuss with their doctors if there was anything to be done to help physically heal the mother, and then they need to decide if and when they will choose to begin trying again. They might even have learned of a genetic disorder that was a precursor to the miscarriage, and that can open a whole other world of decisions for the family plans. All of these discussions contain very private and personal choices to make. When they are ready, and if they choose, they will share their feelings and thoughts with you, and it might open up a conversation at a later time that you can share your wisdom. In the interim though, your job, your *only job*, is to *love them* through their loss and be that quiet shoulder when they need it. It is not *your job* to find an answer for them as to why this happened. And I say this from experience, if you have your own story to share… please be cautious in your timing. It could be incredibly helpful for a grieving couple to know they are not *alone* in their feelings. But try not to use their time as an opportunity to over share your own details; they may not be ready to hear that just yet.

Yeesh, How Long Are You Going To Do This?

This one often made me laugh, because it was truly a sign of lack of education on what all infertility treatments entail. In a world that is very rushed and hurried, and where people are always striving to get everything now, now, now, it is really not that big of a leap for someone to hear you say you are going to do infertility treatments and then turn around six months later and say, "What? You're still doing that?" In this scenario, a little education could go a long way. Primarily, just understanding the nature of infertility treatments, or even the physical miscarriage recovery process, would go far in helping loved ones understand things a little better.

For example, if a couple miscarries a child, it is not a quick process for most. Let's take my own miscarriage as an example. We went for what we believed was an OB appointment to see our baby in September, and found out that the baby was gone. After that, it was a two-month span of time before we could begin even considering to try again. During those two months, we had to complete the miscarriage, wait for my body to heal, and wait for my cycles to begin anew. Definitely not a quick process, and that was *with* us deciding to finalize things with a D & C. Some couples need to wait even longer, depending on the nature of their particular circumstances, and I have met some who had to wait nearly four or six months before trying again. To an outsider, you might hear one day that someone has had a miscarriage and you think how sad you are for them, and you maybe send a card wishing them well. Then a month later you see that person and they have fresh tears from the pain and you wonder, "Wow, still?" Well, to them, that month was still very early on in the reality of the physical ramifications of the loss, much less the emotions. Frankly stated, for most couples, the emotions cannot really be dealt with *until* the physical stuff has found some closure. For me, the two months between September and November was just letting my body heal, and it was not until several months after that I could emotionally find *some* peace with things.

Infertility is another process that is *not* a fast, instant turn around type of deal. Depending on the very unique set of fertility problems a couple encounters, all the treatments are customized to fit and each doctor has their own way of doing things. As such, infertility treatment is not ever a cookie-cutter process. Beyond that, almost all of the month-to-month cycle is dependent on precise timing of the woman's body, financial and work constraints, doctor's timing, and more. In other words, it is precise and calculated and completely out of the control of the actual couple involved. I will use myself again as an example of how wonky and unplanned a "precise and planned" cycle can get. This was one of my more wild and crazy cycles:

- Day 1: Meet with new reproductive specialist and am told we can begin *that day*. Go home with a fist full of prescriptions that you pay for up front.
- Day 2: begin pills for five days.
- Day 4: have proactive HSG procedure "just in case," keep taking pills.
- Day 10: get ready to begin injections, only to be told to stop, HSG found something. Shelve all prepaid prescriptions, start yet new scrip for new hormone and plan surgery.
- Day 20: have surgery (only partially covered by insurance) and begin yet another scrip.
- Day 25: have surgery follow-up and exam and re-begin original plan.
- Day 26: begin more pills for five days.
- Day 31: begin injections.
- Day 36: take different injections and schedule IUI.
- Day 39: do IUI and begin yet another prepaid prescription and begin two-week wait.
- Day 43: do blood test to see if pregnant or not and then lather, rinse, repeat…

The above was *one* cycle. The original plan should have taken twenty-eight days and only cost about twelve hundred dollars. Instead, it took forty-two days and cost around five thousand dollars, and not one thing could have been controlled by us. With that little surgical interruption to our plans, what would have been a short three months of back-to-back treatments at a cost we could afford, was instantly a four or five month process and financial strain we were not expecting. So when someone would ask us how things were going, in a span of a whole month, we could well have *nothing* new to tell them. And this type of "hurry up and wait" approach to medicine is the tip of the iceberg. For couples doing IVF, the regimen and timing is more strict and rigorous, and the ramifications of something going amiss are much larger. A couple could end up prepaying for thousands of dollars in drugs/needles/etc., and then halfway through, the woman could have a cyst that makes them tank the whole cycle, wait thirty days or more, and start over from the beginning.

The true difficulty here for couples struggling is that it is a *daily* process. They *daily* have to take some pill or some shot or attend some doctor's appointment and/or track some bodily function for reporting. Daily. Not weekly or monthly. *Daily*. From their perspective, each and every set back or unexpected cost is a very upsetting and urgent crisis to try and not lose any ground and try to recoup any lost money or precious days. When someone comes along and says, "Yeesh, you're still doing that?" they have no idea that to a couple in the thick of things, you cannot possibly see how slowly things are going. You literally cannot see the forest for all the dang trees! To them, they have only *begun* the process, and knowing that each option could take three to six tries (read three to six months), they could feasibly have *years* ahead of them and still only tipped the iceberg of possibilities. Infertility is not a sprint, it is a long marathon of trial and error. So the next time you see a couple and you think to yourself, "Wow, I cannot believe they are *still* doing that," take a moment to realize that for *that* couple, the end could still be long down the road and they may feel they haven't even begun the journey yet.

Other Erroneous Statements Better Avoided

The above are just a few of the statements heard over and over, but there are surely far more insulting remarks that are not called for in any occasion. I will not go into the detail of explaining why they *could* be construed as helpful or why they should be avoided, but it bears mentioning herein that the below statements are almost *never* okay to say to a couple trying to conceive a child. They all fall under the category of, "Did your mother not teach you that if you cannot say something nice, do not say anything at all?" And, to those of you asking, yes, I have actually heard them all:

- "Wow, do you think you waited too long and your eggs/sperm are too old?" (Yes I do, and thank you for taking note of my futile efforts to rehydrate my decrepit eggs with his ancient sperm.)

- "Have you tried the old-fashioned way?" (*Dang*, I knew I forgot something!)

- "Well, at least you have nieces and nephews!" (Yes, and that totally replaces the need for my own biological child, how could I have missed that little plus.)

- "Hey, you can borrow some of my sperm/eggs if you need it!" (Seriously, this was said. Out loud.)

- "Here, rub my (insert body part) for luck!" (Oh my gosh, why can't the earth swallow me now, or you for that matter.)

- "You're probably better off in this economy to not have a child." (Ah, a good statement from the person who clearly *has* children in this economy.)

- "Don't you have sex enough?" (No comment worth printing…)

These are a few, and there are undoubtedly hundreds more that have been received by other couples going through infertility or pregnancy loss. It is as if people do not realize that not only are these things crass to say in polite company, but likely *dangerous* too. I mean really, if you are talking to a woman who has admitted fertility treatments (pills, shots, patches, etc.) you are taking your life into your own hands by making some of these comments. She's likely sore, hot, hormonal, broke, scared, anxious, and now angry…*At you*!

What Can You Do

If you have read this far into the book (God bless you for it), or have flipped to this page from the table of contents looking for a quick solution, you are likely asking yourself, "What *can* I do to support my loved ones who are struggling with conception difficulties, or who have lost a baby in utero?" Fear not! There are things you *can* do and on behalf of every couple out there who has or is or will be walking this road: *thank you for asking*! As much as there are landmines to avoid, as we discussed above and were shown throughout the biopic portion of this book, there is much that you actually *can* do to show your support and love to someone who desperately needs it. As with just about anything though, timing, tact, and education are the keys. Now for timing/tact, I cannot offer you much. You will learn that on your own, or not, through trial and error. But education can certainly be an area I can help you with. If you did flip to this section and missed the previous fifty thousand words, please do take the time to go back and read from the beginning. It will go far in helping you crawl inside the heart of a hurting couple and understand *why* some things affect those of us dealing with infertility differently than you would expect.

Prior to all our efforts to conceive, if someone told me they were expecting, I would congratulate them, and occasionally ask how they were feeling and attend the baby shower and otherwise not think much upon it. *During* and *after* our struggle, however, I would congratulate them more profusely, ask them how far along they were, and calculate in my mind if they were past the danger zone for miscarriage. I might avoid them on days I was hurting personally, due to a fertility set back, and I would always attend the baby shower with an exit strategy to make a graceful and *early* exit, should I need to. That person would *always* be on my mind with both happiness and sorrow. I would be outwardly happy and inwardly pea green with envy when their birth finally arrived, and I would approach them and their newborns with a sense of awkwardness that I did not know I had in me.

Prior to all our efforts to conceive, if someone told me they had miscarried, I would have likely told them I was sorry and otherwise not thought much upon it. *During* and *after* our own loss, however, I see them with different eyes, and my heart breaks for their pain on a very personal and sympathetic level. I would offer to sit and listen if I could, and might even ask a few questions if I felt they were open to it. I would think of them often, and compare their story to my own to see if they were struggling in familiar territory that I could help with. Their loss would inevitably have me reflecting on my own pain, and I would inwardly weep for us both, if not outwardly weep with them. I would pray for them, of course, and then the next time they did find out they were pregnant, I would hold my breath until they reached the safety zone, knowing full well how possible the chance would be that they would not make it.

Prior to all our efforts to conceive, if someone told me that they were having difficulty conceiving, I would tell them how sorry I was and otherwise say nothing, knowing that in fact I had no education on it. I would likely ask if they had thought about IVF, since it was the key medical term I *did* know, and would undoubtedly make the rookie mistakes that I talk about in this very book. But now, it is a whole different ball of wax. I am forever changed. *Now* if someone tells me they are struggling, I am eager to share with them that we did too, for two-plus years in fact. And I am *eager* to talk with them about their treatments, doctors, options, and specific diagnosis. I have found that often the person I am chatting with is equally eager and relieved to find someone who understands on a basic level what their fears are.

The key here is that prior to all of this, I was just as ignorant and naïve about the ups and downs of infertility as everyone else. But I did not have to be, and neither do you. The fact that you are even reading this book and taking this step shows how much you wish to support someone in your life, and is a huge step in the right direction. But really, if you want to know what you *can* do, this book is not the person to ask. Your *friend* is. Your *loved one* is. Your *spouse* is. Your *coworker* is. The person who motivated you to pick this book up in the first place is your *best* place to start in learning what you can do for them and how. In truth, I do believe that there are blanket things that anyone can do. For example, if you learn that a couple specifically is struggling with an illness like endometriosis or PCOS, then you could easily read up on it and learn a little about the basics. It would take you very little time and would help you to at least understand some of the hurdles they are dealing with, so that if they do talk to you about the various doctor appointments or side effects, you have a better understanding.

But, of all the people in our life who supported us and loved us through our own struggle, my favorite phrase was then (and is now) the one from our friends who said, "I'm sorry you have to go through this and I cannot begin to understand it, but I will pray for you. How specifically can I pray for you *right now?*" That one question would open many doors for me to share, on my own terms, what I needed. And if I was feeling comfortable that day to divulge details, they would listen and comment where they could. If I was feeling more withdrawn and needed to keep it brief, it was my choice to do so. But they were ever-present, always loving and open, and never judgmental. They never doubted our faith or tried to downplay our fears. They never made us feel inadequate or deficient somehow. They never tried to fill the silence with some helpful platitude because of their own awkwardness. They came to us, simply, and shared their sympathy and directly asked what specifically they could pray for at that moment. It was heavenly and simple and wonderful. We knew they cared, but did not feel invaded, and yet if we had a vulnerable moment and needed to talk, they were available and open to it.

Of course, the flip side is the couples that would ignore our situation or us completely. They were uneducated or put off or made uncomfortable, and did not know *how* to support us. So they did nothing. They did not call, they did not e-mail. They did not even make eye contact when they saw us. Or they would call and would chat, but would completely avoid the situation and treat us as if it never happened, and go on and on about *their* lives as if nothing had changed in our own. They would invite us to do things we could not afford to do, and try to include us on things that we could not do because of medical appointments or obligations. They never even acknowledged (either through avoidance or redacted communication) that they were even aware of what we were going through. This was often very painful for us. It somehow made us feel as if we were a burden to them and made them uncomfortable. Often times, I would feel compelled to offer *them* support at a time when I was at my lowest, and then I would feel embittered by it all. After a time, that friendship would inevitably suffer atrophy due to the loss of whatever common ground we once had as friends. Our commonality would get lost in the pile of unspoken sentiments and thoughts. Lost in the feelings hurt and left untended. Engulfed by "the elephant in the room," that everyone ignored.

Ignoring a situation is, in my opinion, never a good or healthy way to go. Granted, you do not have to be more involved than you choose to be. And truly, if a couple's infertility makes you uncomfortable and you cannot be supportive, feel free to find a graceful way to let your friendship take a backseat, so that others may step up and lend a supportive hand. But there is a way to remain in the lives of your infertile friends, even if you do not understand what they are struggling with. Again, the best way to know what you can do, is to simply ask.

The reason I have no pat static answers for you here is simply this: each couple is different. That may sound like an oversimplified statement, but it is very true. Each medical diagnosis is different with diverse side effects, dissimilar causes, unique treatment options, and unequal percentages and chances of success. Each doctor is different in their approach, and thus each couple's individual protocol, or "road to conception," may or may not be alike. And even if you find two couples with identical diagnosis, identical doctors, identical treatments, and identical side effects, you will find two couples that are completely different in their acceptance of their situation. The emotions involved with infertility and pregnancy loss throw a monkey wrench into any one person's efforts to "categorize" a response. A good example of this is the miscarriage I discussed. I miscarried at the same exact time as another couple, and in the same exact manner. I struggled for months to come to grips with the loss, and then grieved in my own way and followed through with a few key things that I needed to do in remembrance of our baby. The other couple grieved in their own way and followed through with their own grief and did their own things in remembrance of their baby. The difference was not only in our manner of grieving, but in how we handled the attempts at conception after that. I re-entered the game fearful, but determined and more motivated than ever to push myself as far as my body or I could go. The other couple re-entered the game more fragile and softly. They grieved the loss longer and needed more time to feel ready to move on. Was their way better or worse than our way? Absolutely not. We each have our own way of grieving a loss and likewise, we each have our own way of dealing with the day-to-day struggles of infertility. Some couples want the anonymous feeling of people *not knowing* what they are going through, so that they can be oblivious and otherwise treated normally. Others need support and prayer and want others to *know* what they are going through. I clearly fell into that second category, *sometimes*. Each couple is unique in their struggle, and their needs are equally unique.

There is a fine line, however, between being supportive and being intrusive. Therein lies the need for tact and timing, two things that I, nor anyone else, can give you. But there are many things that you can talk about that are not overly personal or invasive, but would show you care. Infertility comes with a slew of emotional baggage that we've already discussed, but there is also a ton of practical and logistical hurdles to overcome. Those are often safe areas to open a conversation with to show you care, and then let the other person lead how they feel comfortable. For example, how are they holding up financially? How are they juggling the various doctor appointments with their jobs? Are they able to reorganize some of their financial priorities to accommodate this new goal, or did they need some help/guidance in that area? Was their work supportive or in the dark about what they are trying to do? Have they told their family about their struggles (or if you are family, have they told their friends/church)? These are all vaguely safe areas to inquire that show you care about their well-being, but without being overly invasive if you are unsure where your relationship stands with this person. The next level would be slightly more specific to the closeness of your relationship. How are the medical treatments going? Are you having a hard time with the side effects, or are you physically managing okay? Are you resting/eating well to keep your strength up? Are you able to maintain your normal social calendar, or do you need help with anything? Is your doctor educating you as you go, or have you found information on your own? Do you like your doctor? These fall into the category of someone who has already shared some details of their struggle with you, and you are close enough that you are not being nosy by asking intelligent and pointed questions. Then there is always the really close and personal relationship that can seriously look you in the eye and laughingly ask how your cervical mucus is feeling that day. But if you are close enough to be able to safely discuss that, you certainly do not need a list of Q&A from me!

Some of my most favorite people were the ones who let us talk when we needed to, but otherwise treated us normally and did not avoid us. The couples that would let us know they were praying for us, but did not pry with a slew of invasive questions. The families who would make a note of our next doctor's appointment but not call us daily, wanting to know if "we had heard anything that second." I was never more grateful to my own mother as I was the day that she said, "I always want to know when your pregnancy test is, but I figure if you do not call me with excited news, then it is negative, and the last thing you need is me calling you and digging for painful details." I found out that my mother-in-law and stepmother and one of our close friends were of the same mentality. I loved that! I loved that they cared enough to want to know the big day each month, but were sensitive enough to not pry at a time when I would inevitably be emotional and sad if there was failure on the horizon. You, the reader, can also be a source of infinite love and support, once you learn what it is that your loved one needs. Either your strong silence will carry them through, or your energetic involvement will inspire them to barrel forward. Either your thoughtful actions will send them silent messages of love, or your written cards will send them the love they need in writing when they need it. *Do not be afraid to ask.* "How, specifically, can I pray for you and be here for you right now?" And then do not be afraid to sit back and listen in silence as they share their heart.

Finally, if I were to pinpoint the main thing that I wished my own friends and family had realized when we were going through our struggles, it would be this: infertility is a *whole new world.* A new world that has left its scar on me as a woman, and us as a couple, forever. Not only is your life broken down into its smallest measurements of hours and days, but you begin to celebrate the most minute and asinine things. You have to learn a whole new form of math, and a whole new language of medical terminology and abbreviations along with it. Your life becomes dictated and run by the tyrant of your calendar, and the person who knows you at your most personal level is no longer your friend of ten-plus years, but the nurse at the reception desk of your latest medical specialist. For a long while, Diane, the checkout lady at my RE's office, was my biggest supporter. Your brain is inundated with so many things that *could* or *might* affect the outcome you are working for. Along with the amped up paranoia you are now hyper-aware of the things around you that others take for granted, like easy pregnancies, teen/unwanted pregnancies, abortions, pregnant smokers/drinkers, people doing IVF for fun/convenience, money/job woes, and more. All of this and more is poured into your mind each month, and it truly does change the way you see the world and your place in it. The by-product of which is that it forever, on some level, changes the couple going through it.

Let me repeat that.

Infertility and pregnancy loss will *forever* change the lives of the couple going through it. When you choose, as a couple, to pursue treatment options of any kind for infertility, you are taking your future family that you dreamed of and placing it in the hands of people you *hope* are skilled enough to help you. Obviously it affected me to the point of writing this book, but ask *any* couple who has lost a child to miscarriage or stillbirth, and they will tell you that you never *forget* that baby you loved and lost. You do not *overcome* your grief from the child you will never know. You learn, you cope, you accept, you even move on, but never will you be totally the same as you were before. Infertility is a struggle that is personal and private, and yet life encompassing. Infertility leaves you scrambling for a private place to worry away from your loved ones, while you spread yourself open to your most vulnerable level to strangers. You stress and worry over every dime spent, while willingly shelling out hundreds or thousands of dollars on a chance, a maybe. The logic and illogical co-mingle until your whole world makes little sense and you are swept up in the tide of the daily ride, hoping you can hang on long enough to see it all come to a happy ending. If a couple survives fertility treatments with a baby, they will never *ever* forget what it took to get there, and they will seriously second-guess themselves before trying again. If a couple gets through fertility treatments and decides to adopt or be childless, they will never *ever* forget the cost and heartbreak and loss that led them to that decision. If someone you love is swimming the waters of infertility treatments, they may or may not get to the other shore the way they hope to. Your job, as their support team, is to cheer them on while they struggle, and then pick them up and love them when they falter. The journey is their's alone…but your love and support can make all the difference.

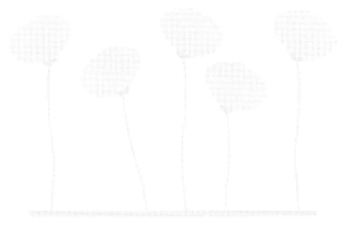

For Warriors in Battle

At the end of the day, there were many things that I learned in our walk that I wished I had known, or had more faith in, up front. I learned so much about myself, my marriage, my friends and family, and my faith. I grew as a person and came out, I believe, stronger for it. But while in the middle of the battle, I could not always see what was right in front of me. Sure, you could tell me I was standing in a forest, but I was still *lost* in the freaking trees! I may not have listened, or even understood it at the time, but I wanted some other couple to tell me they had been there and done that. In fact, that is what inspired this book. I felt sad thinking of other couples out there who were in the trenches of their own battles and could not see *daylight*, much less a friendly face in the battlefield. I did not want even *one* couple to feel they had a scarlet letter sown to their hearts, I did not want even *one* couple to feel as if they had to hide their pain in shame. I wanted to share my story and wisdom with each couple out there and give them hope that even in their *darkest* time, they were not alone on this earth or in heaven. So, for all of you couples going through it right now, whether this sinks in now or later, here are my tidbits of advice and lessons learned that I have saved up just for you.

You Are Not Being Punished

While it is very true that actions and sins have consequences, God is not sitting all high-and-mighty on His cloud and selecting out people for punishment and pain. Quite the contrary. Look through the Bible and you will read of a God who is loving and just and holy and wants nothing more than to be a part of your daily life. God wants to release you of the burden of your sins, and then walk daily with you to show you His loving character. He does not want to sit on the sidelines of your life and watch as you suffer, He wants to gear up and *run that gauntlet with you*. Will He use this as a time to shape you in a way you need? For sure. But at the end of the day, He's not singling you out anymore than He is singling out the other millions of couples struggling at this very moment with any sundry list of illnesses or strains.

As much as infertility can shine a spotlight on your life in a very personal way, it is understandable that you would then turn that spotlight inward and begin to consider things you had not before. But do not let that nagging guilt, that doubt, that fear, add to an already emotional and stressful time. Before you start down that road of beating yourself up for some past sin that you believe has come to haunt you forever, turn to the Bible and embrace God at this time. If you need to confess something that you have been carrying around, then do so, but then accept His eternal forgiveness and allow His love and holiness to wash that burden away. He's not a big, mean God who randomly punishes, so do not think that you are the target of His latest attack. God loves you! Seek help to get healthy in mind, body, and spirit, and let the worry of feeling punished fall to the wayside. It is more of a burden than you need to carry and not worth your time or effort to hold on to.

A Family Is Not a Number, or a Statistic, or a Goal to be Obtained Later

Family is technically defined as a group of people of common ancestry living under one roof. From a social standpoint, however, most people feel that a family is defined as a mom, dad, two kids, and some kind of pet running around. In fact, I myself often felt that we were not a "family" since we did not have kids. My husband would comment on how he loved our little family, and I would usually laugh and crack some joke about all our relatives who lived in different states. But Kevin was right at that time, and I did not see it. We *were* a family, a family of two! I longed and planned and looked forward to all the family traditions we would have when and if we had kids. I would be sad at the holidays to think of how irrelevant decorating a tree was with only two adults in the house. I would get depressed at Thanksgiving or Easter when families would get together for big meals, and we would do what, drive-thru again? Much more emotional pressure was put on my husband and myself on these days due to me missing the entire point that I am now sharing with you.

The important take-away from my cautionary tale is this: a family is what you make of it. Whether it is only you and your spouse or a group of close friends or a church body or a couple of fur-babies in the form of dogs and cats; *that* is your family. You may not fit the uber-traditional mold of two-and-a-half kids and picket fence and a minivan, but you are a family in your own right. If you are not yet pregnant or have a child, that does not make you any less "a family." Instead of sitting around during the holidays mourning the traditions you have yet to begin, relish the time you have with your spouse at that moment and *start* traditions of your own. Yes, infertility is hard and expensive and limiting, but you can still make your own traditions and enjoy the few perks that your life allows as you can. Do not *wait* to begin that Christ-mas ornament tradition for when you can buy "Baby's First Christmas," celebrate each anniversary with an ornament, or each vacation, or some other memorable occasion. When the Fourth of July or Easter or some other occasion rolls around and you begin to feel sad for missing out on some future "family" event, *start now*! Have a Thanksgiving dinner for two; cook it together and enjoy the entire day. If you can, invite over other friends who are in similar situations and make it a group event. If you dream of one day flipping pancakes on Saturday morning for your kids, start now and flip them for your spouse. Enjoy your family, as you have it right now, in whatever way you wish. It will help you to find joy in those small times that will give you hope to carry on when you need it. Heck, I even included our dog in one of our "family photos" for our Christmas card. As far as I was concerned, I had owned my dog longer than I had known my husband, and she was totally my "dog-ter." And to be real here, if you never make it to the finish line of parenthood that you are racing toward, these little traditions will be such *lights* in your world and will give you many wonderful memories to cling to when things get hard. Do not *wait* to be a family when things become perfect. Be one *now*!

The World We Live In Is Often Unfair and Cruel

We've all heard that phrase that life isn't fair. It is so commonplace now that it is used to pretty much excuse just about any behavior these days. As overworked as that statement is (and often times downright irritating too), there is some truth to it. Life is not always fair, and sometimes life often seems like it's out to get you. Please know, that no matter how unfair the world seems right now, it is not because God made it that way, but rather because man inhabits it.

God does not wish for babies to be aborted, or unwed drug addicts to abandon their babies in garbage cans. God does not want that lady outside the grocery store to be smoking while clearly full-term pregnant, nor does he purposefully place these things in your path to taunt you. These things happen in our world because man is sinful by nature and sinful people do sinful things. Or, if you are looking for another good laugh here, stupid is as stupid does. The unfairness that you see is simply amplified by your current circumstances and not because suddenly there is an influx of pregnant people around you. There is no sudden increase, but rather you see it more now. Want to test that theory? Think of a color of car, any car. Think of a bright red car or a lime green car. Think long and hard on that color, and put it in the forefront of your mind. When you get in your own car to drive around, remind yourself that you are thinking of a bright red or lime green car. Now, make a mental note of how many cars you saw that were bright red or lime green. Did the automakers of the world suddenly start selling those colors in rapid succession? Nope. You are more aware of them now, since they are at the forefront of your mind. And that was just a *car*! Think how much more you will notice pregnancy, babies, and the injustices of the world when you are emotionally wrapped up in your own struggle. Of course you will see nothing but babies and bellies everywhere you look when you start each day testing your basal body temperature and end it with an injection of stimulation meds to increase your follicle count. When your day is bookended with fertility, it will seem *filled* with babies and people who you think do not deserve them.

The trick is to not let that feeling torment you. How, you may ask? I have no idea. Sometimes I would verbalize to myself that it was not the world's fault I was infertile. And sometimes I would just get mad and cry. But when that jealous feeling would arise up anew, I would give it to God and that would help me tremendously. You see, God wants all your feelings and emotions and He wants to use them to heal you and help you grow. Do not feel like you have to make your heart perfect and clean and pretty before you open it up to Him. I did not hold back all the horrible things I felt and I would not stifle it down. That helped me a lot and I would encourage you to do the same. Give God your jealousy, your anger, your hurt, your betrayal, *all* of it! Tell Him how upset you are with the smoking pregnant lady. Tell Him how insane the abortion rate is. Tell Him how unfair and horrid your world is, since all your friends seem pregnant and you are not yet. *God can handle it*. Give it up, let it go, and try to find room in your heart for a little grace to the world while you struggle. It will not be easy, and sometimes it might not even be pretty, but if you can manage to let that frustration go it will significantly change your outlook on life. Heck, it might even change your heart a little too.

Open Your Heart to the Children Around You… When You Can

Certainly with infertility, and more so after a pregnancy loss, it is easy to close yourself off to the children in your life. You are hurting and embarrassed and filled with doubts and fears, and the little chubby faces of other people's kids act as tiny reminders of what you do not have. I have been there, I know. There were days I could not face the fact that yet *another* friend of mine was pregnant. I even stopped working in the nursery at church because it was just too hard each Sunday to be surrounded by all those babies and not a single one of them was coming home with me. All those nieces and nephews and kids at church and newborn babies of friends can act like tiny cherubic daggers to your already shredded heart. Do not bury that hurt, but do not indefinitely neglect them your love and attention, either. You may want to shut yourself off and call it "protecting yourself." It seems smart at the time, and you may even rationalize that your friends and family are probably better off without you since it is starting to make them uncomfortable too. To that I say, *Bull*! Instead of avoiding children, embrace them.

If an occasion arises and you have a chance to be around kids, take that moment with them right then, hug them and love them as you would hope to one day have someone love your child. Then, if you need to, give your own pain to God and let Him carry you. Yes, there will be hard days that you need to hide out, it is to be expected, but do not close yourself off to the children in your life completely. Love them, and let God love you through them. After all, "Children are a gift from the Lord; they are a reward from Him" (Psalm 127:3, NLT). Not only will you bless some child with your affection, but you too will be blessed in turn by the innocent and often classic childlike expressions and comments you will receive. You will have a constant reminder of your goal, and a constant source of non-judgmental love given to you in return.

As for worrying about your friends or family being uncomfortable, that is a load of crap! First off, if they truly are uncomfortable, then they need to read this book. It is not their job to feel awkward around you, it is their job to *love you*. You can ease that transition some in how you interact with them, but moreover, you cannot worry about what other people may or may not be feeling by your circumstance. You have *enough* on your plate right now and you need to just let that go.

Fear and Worry Will Paralyze You If You Let It

The worries that come along with a pregnancy loss or infertility, or both, can be absolutely debilitating. I can remember feeling so afraid that I was literally incapable of making a decision. Each month I had a mental list of do's and don'ts, not out of obligation or medical mandate, but fear. So fearful was I that I would allow things in life to pass me by. At one point, I was afraid of *both* continuing on trying to conceive, *and* taking a break and stopping. That is when I knew my worry and fear had reached an uncompromising level that had to stop, and I had to finally let go and let my husband decide what to do.

It is perfectly natural to be worried and afraid when you are dealing with a topic that is so emotionally saturated to begin with. The key is not letting the fear and worry push you too far or drive you to actions, or lack thereof, which are unhealthy and unstable. You have to find a grasp on something solid to keep you grounded during those trying times. For me, I leaned heavily on my husband's level-headed approach to keep from driving us to bankruptcy. I also leaned on the spiritual guidance I received from our pastor, and from the Bible and sermons at church. I would let these *outside* forces act as my grounding corner-stone to keep me level. And finally, when nothing else worked and the fear and worry would overcome me to the point of panicked inaction, I would just…. let go. My husband would pray for me and my pastor would guide me, and I would hand the reins over to cooler heads that I could trust had my best interest at heart.

For me, I could not use one person to lean on; I needed multiple outlets, depending on where my struggle was that day. But whether it is one person for you or a whole team of people, if you do not already have that grounding force in your life, you are *nuts*. Infertility is a crazy ride to be on and if you do not find your center, you will get lost in the ups and downs of it all. Do not think for one second that you will get through something like this without the fear and worry, but instead be prepared and have a support system in place that you can trust to both raise you up when you need it and put you in your place *lovingly* if and when that time comes.

Seek Wise Counsel and Heed Their Advice

Man is not made to be alone and that is never truer than in enduring something as emotionally land mined as infertility. It is easy, and in some ways makes sense, to withdraw and hide yourself from the world. You may even rationalize to yourself that you are withholding personal information that is "no one else's business really." But there is *great* wisdom, comfort, and guidance to be found in Godly counsel, and you are wise to seek it out. Proverbs 11:14 says, "… there is safety in having many advisors." . I believe this is especially true in the fertility struggle that a couple will endure. Think of all the outside influences you will have pulling on you during your infertility journey. You will have medical doctors and specialists telling you what treatment they think you need. You will have pharmacists and drugs dictating your daily life. You will likely have friends, family, and the Internet telling you a host of holistic things you need to be doing. Above all this noise, is your own heart *screaming* at you each day as to how vital and important this dream of parenthood is to you. Your ability to truly tune all that out and discern the right path for you will eventually wear down, and you will *need* some guidance. Finding a spiritual guide to help you discern what God's purpose is for you in all this is vital. It does not have to be your pastor, although I would suggest you go there first. We leaned heavily on our small group for prayer, and then our associate pastor, Pastor Jeff, was integral in giving us the specific guidance we needed during the final year. In the end, Jeff was a *great* source of confirmation that our plan was on the right track. It was *hugely* beneficial to us to have the outside perspective during those trying times.

Psalm 15:22 says, "Plans go wrong for lack of advice; many advisors bring success" . Likewise, Psalm 20:18 says, "… do not go to war without wise advice." Struggling to conceive is certainly a battle of sorts, and it makes sense from a logical and biblical perspective to seek outside, *objective*, spiritual counsel to help keep you on course. These are just a *few* references, whereas the Bible lists many more of them to show that wise counsel is a, well, wise move. With so much pulling at you it is a good decision to seek out an anchor you can lean on when your own judgment becomes clouded by the emotional haze of it all. That person or person(s) can be a source of knowledge you did not know you needed, and moreover, they can and will see things in your journey that you will be blinded to at the time.

Now all of this to say also, be wary of bad counsel. Prayerfully consider who to open yourself to, and be sure that the person or people you choose are prayerful as well. You need someone who will respect your journey and your struggle and will not give you advice based on their own agenda. Instead, you need someone who will guide you based on their own prayerful consideration. Bad counsel is worse than *no* counsel, so seek wisely who you can trust and lean on.

Give Credit When and Where and on Whom Credit Is Due

No matter how strong you think you are, no matter how controlled, organized, efficient, planned, intelligent, or capable you think you are, there will come a time when you come to the end of yourself. The end of your ability to discern where to go or when to stop. The end of your comprehension of your emotional and physical limits. We all have them, and for good reason. But when those times come when you are at the end of yourself, God and likely your spouse and entire support system will be there. They will, as I like to always say, pick you up and put you back together again. They will remind you of who you are and why they love you. They will either help you re-realize your goal to keep going, or they will help you cope with the end of your journey or a break-in your plans. They will support your choices and decisions, they will help you even *make* those decisions at times. And when the dust settles and you regain your footing again, give credit.

Be always thankful to God for his presence, and for the presence of those He has put in your life. Not only is it often humbling to accept the help of others, but it often can bless you in ways unimagined to see how many people love you when you fall apart. I was unforeseeably blessed by just the right people at just the right time. My husband was constant, but I had friends and family and church members who were angels sent to me in need at that exact perfect time. Acknowledge those moments and people when they come. It will help to balance out the times when you emotionally feel sheltered and alone and help you crawl out of yourself enough to appreciate what you *do* have to hold on to.

Pray

You might think to yourself, *Well duh,* but the truth of it is that most people pray only when they are overjoyed or in great, guttering need. They wait until things are blissful and happy and perfect, or bottomed out and they've exhausted all other options. But that is not what God wants with us. God wants to communicate with you daily, and wants you communicating with him *daily.*

Pregnancy loss is a heartbreaking journey and infertility is a unique struggle all its own. With the abundance of emotional ups and downs, not to mention the physical and financial strains, prayer can be a lifeline like no other. Giving God time to communicate with you can renew your spirit on even your darkest day, and uplift you in ways you did not see coming. You probably already know that, but there is more to it. God does not want you to come to Him with only prayerful platitudes that you spout without thought or feeling, he wants *the messy stuff.* How many of us (okay, this is mainly women) hold stuff in, and then one day we blow up completely? Go back and read my chapter on F.U.B.A.R. Friday, and you will see my own example of a time that I let things build and build and finally blew up over the most small and insignificant thing. We often feel that all the small day-to-day things needs to be glossed over or dealt with later, so we do not address them. Then one day, our spouse walks in and knocks over a glass of milk and we go to DEFCON 1, and the war begins.

How often is our prayer life like this? Sure we often pray daily for our daily bread and for general protection, or thanking God for His character, and to be sure these are all good things. But how often do we take the small frustrations to God? How often do we take the small worries and nagging fears to Him? Or more importantly, how many of us take those huge, warring, painful battles to God *first,* instead of our spouse? God does not ask us to come to Him "only when you're clean and happy and ready to honor Him." *No.* God wants us to come to Him *daily,* in every way and in every emotional place we are in at that moment. Feeling great and blessed and lucky? *Great,* take that to God and bless Him for it. Feeling beat down and exhausted and ugly? *Fine,* take that to God and ask Him to show you the beauty in life. Feeling worried and anxious and panic-stricken about the future? *Dandy*, take that to God and ask for His peace and comfort. Worried about the meds, break a nail, get a flat tire, run your panty hose, get a pay cut at work, *anything*, take it to God in prayer and He will use that time to love you in ways you did not know you needed.

But remember this too, *all prayers are heard, but not all are answered in the way we would like or in the time we would wish.* Looking back at my own story, I can see that had God immediately answered my prayer for an instant family, I never would have had the opportunity to grow in my marriage and strengthen my faith, nor even write this book! Perhaps the delays were just time that God was using to mold me into something closer to what He had planned for me. I cannot encourage you enough to pray fervently and daily. Pray knowing that we will *never* fully know His plans for us, but He always *has* a plan for us and will show it in due time.

Respect the Process

In all my time personally, and in all the people I've known in these struggles, this is the one area I wish I could have held on to the most (and helped others hold on to as well). *Respect the process.* It's worth repeating so I'll say it again, **Respect The Process.** The core of this is a startling statistic that I learned. Even the most healthy, normal, fertile couple has, *at best,* a twenty to 30 percent chance to conceive each cycle. There are only two to four days each month that a couple is actually ovulating, fertile, and ready to go, and that is if all other elements are aligned properly, like uterine lining, sperm count and activity, previous relations that month, food and drink effects, and more. Understanding that, really letting that sink in, taught me a lot. For one, it taught me how much of a miracle conception actually is. It is easy to forget that when you hear the startling statistics of teen and unwanted pregnancies that are unplanned, but in truth, each and every conception is a miracle of circumstances that only God could have timed in such perfection. The other thing that this taught me, was that I was *not* going to hit baby pay dirt instantaneously.

Infertility is a process and getting pregnant is not an insta-cure. You do not walk into a clinic, have shots for two weeks and end up instantly pregnant. You must be tested, diagnosed, and learn what specifically needs to happen for your body. This can take several months. Your spouse needs to be tested and diagnosed and see if anything is going on with their body during this time as well. Once that is done, a protocol and plan is set in place to move forward, and that is only if no surgeries or repairs are needed on either you or your spouse. The protocol itself is a guessing game that first month, dependent on how your body reacts. It could take a month or two to level out the meds and find the magic balance *you* need for optimum performance. Once that is found, it can still take three to six months to finally conceive. Keeping all that in mind, a minimum of *one year* of effort should be planned for by any couple going through this process. Does it happen sooner? Sure. Are there couples out there that hit pay dirt on their first go round? You betcha! But if you respect the process and go into it planning on the one year in length, it will help you to not be *so* overwhelmed by the little setbacks that are bound to arise.

For example, perhaps you are being tested and you are fine, but your spouse needs surgery. That could set you back a solid month before you can try again. Or what if you are both ready to move forward, but the drugs have an adverse reaction with your body and you need to start over? That too could set you back month or two getting things leveled back down. Or say that you are both tested, diagnosed, and drugs started, you are still at the mercy of your money, your doctor's schedule, and your bodies timetable. Those are all things you cannot control. Even with all of that in place and ready, you are still facing at least three to six months or more of repetitive trying to find that magic number, that magic cycle, when things finally, hopefully, come together for you. And anytime during that process, you could have other things come up unrelated that put a kink in your plans. Work changes, family crisis, money surprises, and more. If you dive into fertility treatments with the mindset that you will instantly have a baby in your arms, you will be setting yourself up greatly for failure and heartbreak. *Respect* that you are getting the help you need, and respect that if it is going to happen, it will not be on the timetable you planned for.

Your Spouse Is Your Warrior Teammate in Battle

Whether your heart is breaking because of a lost child, or your body is aching from a slew of medical procedures, your spouse is not the enemy. Your husband may be withdrawn in his efforts to deal with this struggle, your wife may be emotional and exhausted, but your spouse is not the enemy. Whether your infertility struggle is one-sided, or both, or neither, *your spouse is not the enemy*. My one constant source of support, no matter my day or mood or need, was my husband. I am forever grateful for his consistency and loving-nature, and the way he carried me through when I needed him to. Moreover though, I have seen many couples that both desperately want to have a baby, but instead of being a team and approaching each day together, they become enemies. The husband does not understand his wife's emotional state, or the wife wishes her husband were more or less emotional than he is. They fight, they argue, they pull at each other, and instead of finding comfort and support on one another, they become adversaries. Remember, you married each other in love and in love you wish to start a family. Do not let that love be buried in hurt feelings and misspoken words.

Wake up folks, *love is a choice*!

If you are resentful of something, talk it out. Maybe you can talk to your spouse, or maybe you need to talk to a pastor or friend or counselor. But never forget that regardless of how this road turns out (with a successful pregnancy or an adoption or neither), your marriage will still be there. It is the cornerstone of your family and should be protected. Do not let the finances, the drugs, the doctors, the stress, or the worry become a wedge between you. Rather, the two of you should become a fortress together to battle these things as they arise. Let the waters of doubt crash against as you stand strong together, with God completing your team. And when in doubt, when you look at your spouse and they seem wholly unlovable, remember that you too were once that way, and God loved you still. *That* is the example that has been set countless times for us to follow. Not a love of passion or emotion or moment, but an active love that is chosen day by day, again and again. Just read Corinthians 13 to get a rundown of the tougher side of love, the one that "bears all things" and is not "easily provoked." *That is* the hard love that you will be faced with during these trying times. Making your spouse the enemy will only isolate you both further and make the struggle all that much more difficult. But finding that active love that God has demonstrated will make things much easier on you both and will make a world of difference in your marriage as a whole.

Blame and Bitterness Will Ruin Your Marriage, If You Let It

This is a big one that I was blessed to not struggle too much with myself, but that I saw other couples really get beat up over. Blame is a deadly and slippery slope upon which your marriage could be irreparably damaged. It is easy to fall into and a great tool for the Devil to use as a wedge between you. No matter how much a couple wants a baby, and no matter how unified they may feel at the onset of their struggle, at some point, a doctor will test you both to determine what the hurdle is that needs to be overcome. Maybe you and your spouse will be like my husband and I. We both had issues. But more likely, you have only one of you that needs the assistance. Perhaps the husband does not have a high count or quality to his sperm. Perhaps the wife does not ovulate or has scarring in her tubes blocking the way. Or, even more heart-wrenching, maybe you are both fine and it is unexplained infertility.

It is almost effortless, once the drugs start and the disappointments and failures pour in upon you, to look at the wounded and broken spouse and blame them for your pain. It is so simple to look at your husband, who has zero sperm count, and be bitter and angry at your own need for all these drugs because he is deficient in your mind. It is easy to look at your wife, who has scarred tubes and cannot ovulate, and blame her for the high medical cost and emotional ups and downs. It is almost expected to look at yourself, who has just miscarried yet another baby, and feel that there must be something wrong with you to keep having this happen. It is so easy to do and it will so easily *ruin* you both. *There is no winning in the blame war.* There is no purpose for it, no possible reason to justify it, and no goal to be obtained by it. There is absolutely nothing good that will come out of blame other than your own bitterness, which becomes a catalyst for problems all it's own.

Let me repeat that. There is *no good* that comes from blame.

If you do find yourself looking at your spouse with contempt and anger, immediately, *right then,* get on your knees and give it to God. Do not wait until it festers and grows, do not delay until you lash out in a weak moment and hurt them. *Confess* your heart to God, and ask Him to help you set aside your selfish feelings for the sake of loving your spouse the way He commanded you to. If you still struggle after that, continue to pray, but go and seek out support in the form of a pastor or trusted mentor/friend. *Get* the support you need and the outlet you need to be able to really get to the root of what your blame and bitterness is about. And when all else fails, look at the example that Jesus gives us about loving forgiveness and unconditional care. Jesus was sent here on this earth to *die* for us, all of us. And how have we behaved and treated that gift? Do we deserve it? No. Does He love us unconditionally, despite all our flaws and shortcomings? Absolutely. And that tall order is the example He has laid at our feet to follow. We are to love our spouses unconditionally, even if we do not think they are very lovable at that moment.

Cherish the Moments of Rare Bliss in Your Life That Surprise You

When you are on the journey through infertility and struggling to heal from a lost pregnancy, it is easy to dismiss the little moments of happiness that do occur. It could be as simple as a cup of coffee on a Saturday morning with your spouse that leads to *great* conversation and easy laughter. Or it could be a birthday that you actually have the *money* to really celebrate and do a weekend trip together. Either way, do not let those moments pass with a bittersweet taste. Instead, try to set aside the struggle, the hurt, the worry, the fear, for just that moment. Embrace that moment as a blessed gift from God, a reprieve from the drudgery. For those moments, often too few and far between, will give you so much release that you did not know you needed.

Laughter and joy can be healing if you let them, and even that small laugh over a cup of coffee with your spouse can help to heal potential hurt feelings or bolster up the reserves of love you have for one another. A celebrated birthday can help to remind you that *yes,* you may be childless now, but you have *much more* to love, and that makes your life rich and meaningful. Do not let these moments come with a tinge of guilt or pain; embrace them and milk them for all they are worth!

At the End of the Day

When push comes to shove, infertility is a journey. Miscarriage is a process. Nothing is instant in our instant world. The more we can cling to God and to each other during difficult times, the more we can surf the waves as they hit and enjoy the calm waters when they arrive. My journey was not only one of family efforts to conceive, but a journey that ultimately strengthened my marriage, my faith, my endurance, and more. Regardless of the outcome, Kevin and mine's ability to cling to God and one another through the harsh realities and struggles was, and is still today, the truest of rewards.

Losing a child, or being told you will never have a child, is definitely one of the greater heartbreaks that a couple will endure. But it is certainly not the only one and, most especially, not the biggest one. God can and will use these trials to strengthen you in ways you did not think possible. All you have to do is let Him in, and let go of your other plans.

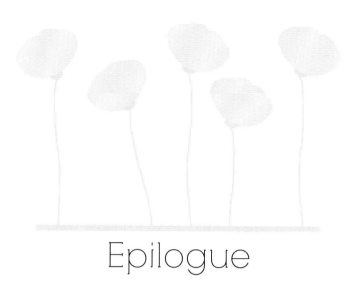

Epilogue

Before I could call this little project of mine completely finished, I simply had to share some wisdom that I had gleaned from our trials to other couples going through this. I mean, of all the things I might have wanted to do with this book, the very top of the list was to help other couples out there feel less alone in their walk. Infertility is, at the very best of days, a whipping and a half! The physical and emotional damage inflicted on our bodies and minds is enough to beat anyone down spiritually, and considering how taboo the topic still is in society, it is no wonder that most people going through it need antidepressants and counseling just to survive it. I could have dedicated this entire portion of my book to couples as a whole, but I felt more inclined to rather speak to only the women out there. Likewise, my husband has generously offered up his insight to the men involved. Our hope is that by addressing you individually, our advice will be better received and understood. Our hope, is that your marriage survive infertility and pregnancy loss not only intact, but stronger than ever. We firmly believe that God will guide you in this process if you let Him. We also firmly believe that as husbands and wives, there are things we can and cannot do to help this along. So without further ado…

A Note to Wives

In scripture it tells us to:

> [21]And further, submit to one another out of reverence for Christ. [22] For wives, this means submit to your husbands as to the Lord. [23] For a husband is the head of his wife as Christ is the head of the church. He is the Savior of his body, the church. [24] As the church submits to Christ, you wives should submit to your husbands in everything.
>
> *Ephesians 5:21–24*

If you are like me, this scripture holds a lot of difficult pills to swallow. I was raised by a single mother, and between her living example and society's standards, I was given, time and time again, an example of what *strong,* independent women were supposed to be like. The ideal was shown to me in being that of a charismatic, beautiful, dominant force of nature type of being. Loners? Perhaps. Everything to everybody? Maybe. But in all things I learned, either by example or words or both, that *men* were never to be something that controlled me or ran my life or guided my decisions. The word *submission* was perverted into a description of weakness. It still carries, for me, a sense of domination and controlling influence and as such, I cringe to hear it even to this day. But that was *not* how this verse was intended to be read, and if you stop with *that* verse, you are missing the beauty of what the Lord intended for marriages. My husband addresses the portion of scripture dedicated specifically to men, but the end of it all states the following:

> [31]As the Scriptures say, "A man leaves his father and mother and is joined to his wife, and the two are united into one." [32] This is a great mystery, but it is an illustration of the way Christ and the church are one. [33] So again I say, each man must love his wife as he loves himself, and the wife must respect her husband.
>
> *Ephesians 5:31–33*

The subtext of these verses is not "Men, rule over your wives with an iron hand and ladies, don those aprons and get back into the kitchen.

HEATHER D. NELSON

Kick your shoes off, birth the babies, and keep your yap shut!" The real message to all this is simply that husbands and wives are to *forever* love and respect each other. Men have their own struggles in this, but for us wives, I believe there is a key relevance to this in regards to family planning, infertility, and the loss of a pregnancy.

Simply put: infertility, and the emotional state it can place you in, is *no excuse* for walking over your husband like a doormat.

That might seem harsh to read, but in case you have not noticed, I am not one to mince words. Marriage is a beautiful thing and, when running as God intended, is a well-oiled machine of support and laughter and bonding and togetherness that can withstand anything the world can throw at you. Never in my own life have I needed that machine to run properly as I did when my body and heart were simply chewed to pieces in the face of infertility and the loss of my dear Peanut. I cannot even fathom how much *more* difficult my life would have been had I not had the unending support and love of my husband, and I know that he would not have felt as free to *give* me that support and love had I chosen to walk all over him. A woman is a beautiful creature that God has gifted with a world of emotional capacity. We can love so deeply and in turn, be hurt or brokenhearted just as passionately. It is easy, and almost expected in this society, to lash out at those closest to us when our reserves of emotions runs dry. In fact, how often have we been forced to put on a brave face at work, or church, or the grocery store, never *daring* to be rude to a stranger or impolite to a coworker, only to come home and feel no shame at snipping at our husbands. We often assume that because he loves us, and we are married, that he will not only *understand* our emotional fragility, but accept it freely when we decide to berate him endlessly about some small perceived slight. I speak of experience here ladies, my own husband has had to remind me on several occasions that in my stress and frustration, I had become less than kind to him in my words and actions.

So to all the wives out there I say, "*Get over yourself!*"

Infertility is hard not only for us, but for our husbands as well. Men may handle and process the stresses of the journey differently from us, and at times they might even seem shut down or mentally checked out, but that does not ever give us the right to be hurtful or hateful to them. Our husbands, who we loved enough to marry and vow our lives to, deserve our *respect,* even when we are, ourselves, at our lowest. You may ask, "What is respect exactly?" Well, that is an easy question to answer. The dictionary describes respect, among other things, as a place of high regard and high esteem. For me, that means that my husband is not "some close friend I can browbeat in my difficult times, expecting him to take it," but rather that my husband is someone I should love, honor, and cherish all the days of my life. Does that ring a bell? Let me say that again. Your husband is deserving, *everyday*, of your love and honor. Or better yet, backup your reading in Ephesians to a few key versus that lead into this:

> [15]So be careful how you live. Do not live like fools, but like those who are wise. [16] Make the most of every opportunity in these evil days. [17] Do not act thoughtlessly, but understand what the Lord wants you to do. [18] Do not be drunk with wine, because that will ruin your life. Instead, be filled with the Holy Spirit, [19] singing psalms and hymns and spiritual songs among yourselves, and making music to the Lord in your hearts. [20] And give thanks for everything to God the Father in the name of our Lord Jesus Christ.
>
> *Ephesians 5:15–20*

What I pull from that is that I should make the most of *every* day I have with my spouse. I should be always thoughtful of him and be filled with joy when I think of him. I should thank God each and every day for my blessings, chief amongst them being my husband.

I should always be careful not to let my emotions run my husband or myself into the ground. This is often hard, as a woman, to do and even more so with all the stresses of infertility and pregnancy loss. Our hearts get so wrapped up in the struggle that we forget *why* we are struggling. We are not *just* trying to have a baby, ladies, but grow our *family!* My husband has often stated that the best gift he could ever give our children is to love their mother. I kind of laughed at that at first, but the more I thought about it, the more I realized I could learn a little bit from my husband's insight. How much more would my own children learn about how to be *better* adults in their own lives, than to see the example that I had set in my own home?

In the end, it would never matter how much we struggled and strived and wanted a baby, if our marriage fell apart to achieve it. How much better to get to the end of our road and still have our husbands, our mates, our best friends, our life partners by our side, stronger than ever! I cannot speak on behalf of my husband directly, but I can tell you as a wife, that I see far more loving reactions from him when I first *show* him the respect and love he deserves. Let me leave you ladies with one more bit of scripture that I really find comforting and often convicting at the same time.

[1] If I could speak all the languages of earth and of angels, but did not love others, I would only be a noisy gong or a clanging cymbal. [2] If I had the gift of prophecy, and if I understood all of God's secret plans and possessed all knowledge, and if I had such faith that I could move mountains, but did not love others, I would be nothing. [3] If I gave everything I have to the poor and even sacrificed my body, I could boast about it; *but if I did* not *love others, I would have gained nothing.*

[4] Love is patient and kind. Love is not jealous or boastful or proud [5] or rude. It does not demand its own way. It is not irritable, and it keeps no record of being wronged. [6] It does not rejoice about injustice but rejoices whenever the truth wins out. [7] Love never gives up, never loses faith, is always hopeful, and endures through every circumstance.

[8] Prophecy and speaking in unknown languages and special knowledge will become useless. But love will last forever! [9] Now our knowledge is partial and incomplete, and even the gift of prophecy reveals only part of the whole picture! [10] But when full understanding comes, these partial things will become useless.

[11] When I was a child, I spoke and thought and reasoned as a child. But when I grew up, I put away childish things. [12] Now we see things imperfectly as in a cloudy mirror, but then we will see everything with perfect clarity. All that I know now is partial and incomplete, but then I will know everything completely, just as God now knows me completely.

[13] Three things will last forever—faith, hope, and love—and the greatest of these is love.

1 Corinthians 13

When you struggle in your journey to have a baby, when you grieve for the loss of a child you never held, when the medical stresses and financial woes become too much for you to bear, do not lash out at your husband and be hateful, disrespectful, or cruel. *Lean* on him and open your heart to him and remember that your husband is in this too. *With you,* not *against you.* If you show him respect always, and he gives you the love you need, you can *never* fail. I pray that each and every one of you, as women, find the balance that you need during difficult times and the love you so deserve!

A Note To Husbands: by Kevin Nelson

Whenever I consider my role as a husband, I always go to Ephesians 5:25: "Husbands, love your wives, as Christ loved the church and gave himself up for her" (NIV). This scripture verse is loaded, and it is probably the inspiration for many books on marriage. Even though it may be nothing new, I want to focus briefly on three things that this verse tells me about my role as a husband, and share how this has related to our struggles with fertility.

Love Your Wife Unconditionally

The first thing that Ephesians 5:25 tells me about my role as a husband is that I need to love my wife unconditionally. Christ has loved me through thick and thin, when I least deserve it, and even when I have completely rejected him. No matter what I have done, Christ has always been there with open arms to receive me back whenever I am ready to turn around. If I am to love my wife in this same way, then I cannot perceive anything that she could possibly do that would warrant me to stop loving her.

One day during our struggle, my wife called up the associate pastor at our church and asked him to come over to pray with us about the infertility. There was no real "reason" to do this, other than she just felt we needed it. When the pastor arrived, instead of the quick fifteen minute chat and prayer that we expected, he spent hours with us, probing to see where each of us was at, and finally offering some advice. In our case, I had faith and trust that God would give us a baby in His time and that, even if he did not, things would still work out. My wife, whose life's aspiration was to be a mother, had a much harder time with this particular crisis. Our pastor suggested that this might be a good time for her to "ride my coattails." He gave the example of a ship's icebreaker that does the job of breaking the ice for other ships, and suggested that she allow me to fill a similar role throughout this struggle. I believe his exact words to me were, "You need to step up!" Prior to our family plans, my wife had been afraid that if she was too needy, I might decide that our marriage was too difficult and leave her. This was an undo amount of pressure she had on herself. After this conversation with the pastor, she allowed herself to lean on me more, and as a result of my stepping up to the task at hand, she ended up with a stronger security and a deeper respect for our marriage.

I asked my wife what actions specifically told her that I loved her unconditionally. The first example she could think of was when I would mix-up the fertility drugs and give her the shots. This seems like such a small and insignificant thing, but that simple action told her I loved her, that we were going through the journey together, and that I was helping in the only way that I could. I do not know what actions will tell your wife that you love her. However, you can start with simply telling her. Let your wife know that she can lean on you. Then, find small ways to show that love by working together as a team. Or as my wife likes to say, "Take this opportunity to man up."

When facing the struggles of infertility, the last thing your wife should have to worry about is whether you still love her and will continue to love her through infertility struggles. She should have the peace of mind that no matter how hard things get, the one thing that she can always rely on is your love and support. So, make sure that your wife knows you love her and will do so unconditionally forever.

Love Your Wife Sacrificially

The second thing that Ephesians 5:25 tells me about my role as a husband is that I need to love my wife sacrificially. Christ was fully God and fully man. Being fully man, I believe that Christ had the same human desires that most of us have, to have a wife, to have children, to be successful, to live a long life. Even at the end of His life, we see Him asking the Father if there was any other way that He would not have to sacrifice Himself on the cross (Matthew 26:36–44). However, He sacrificed His earthly desires in order to fulfill His godly purpose, which was to redeem mankind. If I am to love my wife in the same way, then I need to put her needs before my own. Never is this truer than during the loss of a child or the struggle to become parents with infertility difficulties.

Loving your wife sacrificially does not mean that all you do is whatever she wants you to do. You do not have to become a doormat to live a godly life. Rather, loving your wife sacrificially is done with deliberate choices to put off something that you want to do in order to fulfill a need in the life of your wife. For instance, let's take the following scenario. On Friday nights, you have a night out with the guys, and you've been looking forward to it all week. However, when you get home from work you find that your wife has had a rough day and really needs to talk to you about it. The choice goes through your head: tell her that you will talk to her when you get home, or call the guys and tell them that you cannot make it. What do you do?

I do not really have any formula for knowing how and when to sacrifice your own plans for the sake of your wife's needs. Sometimes it may be a choice for a onetime event. At other times, it may be a change to your schedule or budget on an ongoing basis. For one person, it may be giving up a single night with the guys to have a night spent supporting his wife. In my case, since I had a flexible work schedule, I tried to go to every doctor's appointment where there was anything invasive (which turned out to be most of them), so multiple times per week. On those days, I worked late those evenings but was at least present for the appointments in the daytime. For others who might not have that kind of flexibility, it may simply mean setting up some more structure in the

HEATHER D. NELSON

schedule—date nights, etc.—that provide opportunity for their wives to vent. Also, I made sure that our budget allowed for weekly dates for the two us, and the periodic pedicure for my wife. She really looked forward to those little splurges and they were often highlights to her week.

I imagine that most of us know when we are being selfish and when we are being selfless. The hardest part about giving sacrificially is not in understanding it, but in *overcoming* our own desires to make ourselves happy first, and only making other people happy insofar as it benefits our own happiness. I think it goes without saying that all of us, myself at the top of the list, can love our wives more than we do and could afford to give a little more sacrificially than we do, in order to show our wives how much we love them. When your wife is going through the physical and emotional rigors of infertility and pregnancy loss, this is a *great* opportunity for you to explore your more selfless side.

Love Your Wife Proactively

The third thing that Ephesians 5:25 tells me about my role as a husband is that I need to love my wife proactively. When Christ died for our sins, the human race did not even know that it needed a Savior. We thought we could live a mostly good life, make the good outweigh the bad, and if we succeed in that, we get eternal bliss in heaven. We did not ask Him to sacrifice Himself, the thought never would have crossed our minds. In fact, most of us would prefer to "earn" our way into heaven, so that it is something that we accomplished rather than coming to terms with being a sinner that is not worthy of heaven on our own, but only made worthy by His grace. However, despite our resistance to Him, Christ knew our needs and took care of them. If I am to love my wife in the same way, then I will proactively seek out my wife's needs and try to fulfill them without having to be asked for everything.

Now, I will be the first to tell you that this is probably my biggest weakness. My nature is to go about my own routine with my blinders on and only help out after my wife specifically asks me to help. In fact, just today, my wife got frustrated with the fact that she had to ask for my help with the baby when we are getting ready for church on Sunday mornings. I get myself ready and just leave her to do the rest. Part of this is from the fact that five days out of the week, my only job is to get myself ready for work, but the rest is from me not being proactive.

Being proactive means getting to know your wife. In getting to know her, you will see the things she needs. Through the infertility struggle, for instance, I observed that my wife was stressed out, which, oddly, did not require any special skills of observation on my part. But more than just "stressed out," I observed that she would specifically stress out about the house not staying clean. In trying to be proactive, I had some choices. I could give the ultimate in loving sacrifice and try to clean the house myself, which would probably take me twenty hours a week, leave the house messy, and leave me stressed out too (I am the slowest house cleaner the world has ever known). Alternatively, I could give a little less sacrificially and just budget for someone to clean the house. I am notoriously tight with a buck, so it was a sacrifice on my part, but not a huge sacrifice by any means, and it helped meet Heather's needs immensely.

You do not have to be omniscient like God and know all of your wife's needs before she even asks. It is perfectly acceptable, and advisable, to ask your wife what you can do to help her. When you ask your wife if she has any needs, that is still being proactive. However, there are some things that your wife will need that she will not even know herself. It may be that you will actually see how stressed out she is before she sees it herself. That is why it is important to be observant and proactive. And the key here is that when you discover something that your wife needs, *fill that need.*

Going through fertility treatments can be a rough journey. I would like to be able to give you the perfect solution to everything, but everyone's journey is different. Most of this journey will need to be figured out by lots of open and honest communication between you and your wife, and do not forget, lots of prayer for wisdom and guidance. However, there are a few things that I consider important and would like to mention as potential practical tips that may help someone, somewhere, to perhaps avoid some pitfalls. So, here is my short list of advice.

Avoid Debt

My wife and I were fortunate that we went through Dave Ramsey's class, Financial Peace University, and were able to get rid of most of our debt before we got too far into the pricier fertility treatments. Aside from alleviating our debt, going through Dave Ramsey's class also put us on the same page financially. Being united in our goal to avoid debt, and having ourselves mostly free of debt, opened the door for us to pay cash for all of the doctor's visits, injections, and IUIs. Avoiding going into debt for the fertility treatments kept us from adding that stress to an already stressful situation.

You cannot put a price on having a baby. However, with fertility treatments, there are no guarantees. In my personal estimation, the most important thing to consider is your marriage. It will do you no good to succeed in having a baby, only to find that your marriage has broken apart because of financial stress. More importantly, in the event that fertility treatments are unsuccessful, you will need each other to lean on. Therefore, you need to make sure you keep your marriage on the forefront of your decisions. In that light, before you go into any debt for fertility treatments, I would encourage you to do the following:

- If you have existing debt, seriously consider working to get out of debt prior to fertility treatments. I highly recommend Dave Ramsey's seven steps in Financial Peace University.

- If you do go into debt, do not go into any debt that you are not okay having, even if the treatments do not succeed.

- If either you or your wife are not okay with debt, do not do it. The last thing you want is the treatments not to work, and then the spouse that wanted no debt to be bitter about it.

- Absolutely, you and your wife should work to agree on every decision you make. This is a team effort. If you do not agree, spend time in prayer, and get a third party (counselor, pastor, etc.) to help mediate the discussion as needed.

I've heard it said a number of times that the leading cause of divorce is financial problems. I do not know how true that is, and in some cases, I think "financial problems" is a mask for other deeper issues. However, the one thing that I do know is that adding that kind of financial stress on to an already stressful situation is something that I think you should avoid if at all possible.

Consider it carefully. Consider it prayerfully.

Take What Stress You Can From Your Wife

Everyone is different. Some husbands may be good at doing housework and may help their wife in that way. I suck at housework, so I hired someone to come once a week. Another thing that I did was tried to keep the "financial stress" away from my wife. If we were getting a little tight and I was stressing about it, I tried to keep my own stress away from her as much as possible.

The main thing is to try to find some things that you can do that can help relieve some of the worries and stresses your wife might have. Whether that is the grocery shopping, the laundry, or something else you think you can do for her, just try to do *something* to let your wife know that you are in this journey *with* her.

Be Affectionate and Understanding (Non-Sexually)

If you're going through anything beyond IUI, your wife is likely getting poked and prodded multiple times per week. This will leave her feeling very non-sexual and often unattractive too. However, she still needs to know that you love her, but without the pressures to be more sexual than she is comfortable being. Be generous in your non-sexual affections to help reassure her of your love, and to maintain your closeness even in times when you cannot be physically intimate. Always be honest with your needs, but do not pressure or push her to go beyond what she is willing and able to do. And no matter what goes on in the bedroom, hugs and kisses should be given freely throughout the day to bolster up that love tank for your wife.

People Can Be Stupid, Protect Your Wife

Unfortunately, many people out there say stupid and hurtful things. Whether it is saying that you do not have faith in God by going through fertility treatments, asking why you do not just adopt, or just coming up and constantly asking if you're pregnant yet, these things can be an irritation at best, and often hurtful to your wife. Many of them are well-meaning people that do not have a clue what you are going through but feel that they need to say something.

If you can, try to run interference for your wife. My wife really appreciated it one day when I saved her from some ladies I knew she was trying to avoid. All I did was walk over, told them that I was sorry to interrupt, but that I had to get my wife to lunch, and then I started walking and dragging my wife along. Honestly, I do not even remember this story, but my wife does, and in her estimation, I am a hero for it. If you can, find out if there are any particular people that your wife would like you to help her avoid, and if you see the vultures start flying around her, swoop in and save the day. Be warned, it could be *family* who is hurtful. You will need to always practice tact and respectful intervention, but mastering this will bring you *big* husband points with your wife!

Be a Team

Whether fertility issues are on the husband's or wife's side, the wife is the one who gets to have her body the most invaded. My wife often described the physical rigors of infertility treatments as equivalent to running out in the street to be hit by a car, then handing the driver five hundred bucks and thanking them and asking them if they'd like to return next month and do the same thing again. It is no walk in the park, from what I understand. Therefore, I would like to encourage husbands to bend over backward a little bit to try to show your wife that you are committed to the process, committed to her, and by her side—working as a team.

That said, unless your wife is very different from mine and does not want you to go to her doctor's appointments, go to as many of the medical appointments as you can, particularly the ones that are more invasive. Just being there with her, by her side, can be a huge communication that the two of you are a team. If you have to pick and choose, then in my estimation, the most important appointment to be at is the insemination or implantation (with IUI or IVF, respectively). Thereafter, it would probably be the sonograms where they check follicle growth, etc., since that is also invasive.

I realize that not all husbands have a flexible schedule to be able to do this. So, in that case, try to let your wife know that you are both on the same team, shooting for the same goal, in whatever way you can. Whether that is mixing up the injections and giving them to her, setting up some extra dates throughout the week to help her unload, rubbing her feet while you watch television, or whatever else you can do to help her.

If you focus on your marriage as your number one priority and walk through this journey together, then I am confident that you will come out the other side stronger than you went in.

> Two are better than one,because they have a good return for their work:
> If one falls down,his friend can help him up.
> But pity the man who falls and has no one to help him up!
> Also, if two lie down together, they will keep warm. But how can one keep warm alone?
> Though one may be overpowered, two can defend themselves.
> A cord of three strands is not quickly broken.
>
> *Ecclesiastes 4:9–12 (NIV)*

HEATHER D. NELSON